Clinical Nutrition in Practice

Clinical Supervision in Practice

Clinical Nutrition in Practice

Nikolaos Katsilambros, MD
Charilaos Dimosthenopoulos, MMedSci, SRD
Meropi Kontogianni, PhD
Evangelia Manglara, SRD
Kalliopi-Anna Poulia, MMedSci, AssocNutr

Athens University School of Medicine
Laiko University Hospital
Athens
Greece
&
Department of Nutrition and Dietetics
Harokopio University
Athens
Greece

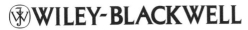
WILEY-BLACKWELL

A John Wiley & Sons, Ltd., Publication

This edition first published 2010
© 2010 Blackwell Publishing Ltd

Blackwell Publishing was acquired by John Wiley & Sons in February 2007. Blackwell's publishing programme has been merged with Wiley's global Scientific, Technical, and Medical business to form Wiley-Blackwell.

Registered office
John Wiley & Sons Ltd, The Atrium, Southern Gate, Chichester, West Sussex, PO19 8SQ, United Kingdom

Editorial offices
9600 Garsington Road, Oxford, OX4 2DQ, United Kingdom
2121 State Avenue, Ames, Iowa 50014-8300, USA

For details of our global editorial offices, for customer services and for information about how to apply for permission to reuse the copyright material in this book please see our website at www.wiley.com/wiley-blackwell.

The right of the author to be identified as the author of this work has been asserted in accordance with the UK Copyright, Designs and Patents Act 1988.

Wiley also publishes its books in a variety of electronic formats. Some content that appears in print may not be available in electronic books.

Designations used by companies to distinguish their products are often claimed as trademarks. All brand names and product names used in this book are trade names, service marks, trademarks or registered trademarks of their respective owners. The publisher is not associated with any product or vendor mentioned in this book. This publication is designed to provide accurate and authoritative information in regard to the subject matter covered. It is sold on the understanding that the publisher is not engaged in rendering professional services. If professional advice or other expert assistance is required, the services of a competent professional should be sought.

Library of Congress Cataloging-in-Publication Data

Clinical nutrition in practice / Nikolaos Katsilambros . . . [et al.].
       p. ; cm.
    Includes bibliographical references and index.
    ISBN 978-1-4051-8084-9 (pbk. : alk. paper)   1. Dietetics–Miscellanea.   2. Diet therapy–Miscellanea.
I. Katsilambros, Nicholas.
    [DNLM: 1. Nutrition Disorders–Handbooks.   2. Nutrition Therapy–Handbooks.   3. Nutritional
Physiological Phenomena–Handbooks. WD 101 C641 2010]
    RM217.C65 2010
    615.8′54–dc22

                                                                                              2010007725

A catalogue record for this book is available from the British Library.

Set in 10/12 pt Avenir by Aptara Inc., New Delhi, India
Printed and bound in Malaysia by Vivar Printing Sdn Bhd

1   2010

Contents

Preface

Nutrition is of central importance to the treatment of various diseases and health conditions, just as malnourishment is largely responsible for their prevalence. In recent decades, great emphasis has been placed on the importance of nutrition and a healthy diet, especially in hospital settings, since malnutrition is a widely presented problem and an appropriate dietary plan can shorten the treatment period and hence the duration of a patient's hospitalisation.

Clinical Nutrition in Practice is aimed at health professionals who are involved in the general medical treatment of patients. The book is in the form of questions and answers, in order to be more interesting and practical for the reader. It contains short answers on topics related to different scientific fields of nutrition, based on the recent literature, and can be used as a scientific tool for all professionals in daily practice.

I would like to thank all the authors of the book, who are clinical dietitians and nutritionists with great experience in the clinical field, with whom I collaborated on a daily basis, in 'Laiko' General Hospital, Athens, Greece. I would like especially to thank Charilaos Dimosthenopoulos (RD) for his cooperation in the general organisation of the book.

I would also like to thank Wiley-Blackwell for publishing this book. It has been a great honour to work with them on it, and I hope that it will extend and deepen health professionals' knowledge and understanding of clinical nutrition.

Professor Nikolaos Katsilambros
MD, PhD (Athens University), FACP

Chapter 1

Principles of Healthy Nutrition

Charilaos Dimosthenopoulos, Meropi Kontogianni and
Evangelia Manglara

Energy balance

What is energy balance?

Energy balance is the difference between energy intake, which can be metabolised, and total energy expenditure. It could be said that the human body's energy state is balanced when its energy expenditure is equal to its energy intake.

The human body requires energy to perform its many functions, to facilitate muscle activity and developmental demands and to correct problems that may have been caused by disease or injury. Energy needs are met by the energy obtained from the body's diet, which derives from foods either of plant or of animal origin. Food energy is released in the body through the oxidation of carbohydrates, fats, proteins (which are called macronutrients) and alcohol.

If energy intake and expenditure are not equal, the result will be either a positive energy balance, in which body energy stores (and mainly fat) are increased, or a negative energy balance, in which the body falls back on using its energy stores (fat, protein and glycogen). Consequently, the body's energy balance (along with other factors) determines to a large extent its weight and general health status.

What factors influence how much energy the human body requires?

According to the definition given by the World Health Organization (WHO), energy requirement is 'the level of energy intake that will balance energy expenditure when we have a body size and composition, and a level of physical activity consistent with long-term good health'. Energy requirements are influenced by various factors, such as the developmental stage we are in (e.g. children's or adolescents' requirements are different from those of the adults), body size, the amount and intensity of physical activity (athletes and manual workers, for instance, obviously require more energy than people doing clerical work or leading sedentary lives), gender, illness, injury, pregnancy, lactation, etc.

What is the basal metabolic rate?

The basal metabolic rate (BMR) is one of the three components that energy expenditure consists of. It is the amount of energy spent for basal metabolism, which represents voluntary and involuntary vital bodily functions, such as respiration, renal, brain and cardiovascular functions, cell and protein turnover, blood circulation, the maintenance of body temperature, etc.

BMR is commonly extrapolated to 24 hours to be more meaningful, and it is then referred to as 'basal energy expenditure' (BEE), expressed as kcal/24 h (kJ/24 h). Resting metabolic rate (RMR), energy expenditure under resting conditions, tends to be somewhat higher (10–20%) than under basal conditions owing to increases in energy expenditure caused by recent food intake (i.e. by the thermic effect of food) or by the delayed effect of recently completed physical activity. Thus, it is important to distinguish between BMR and RMR and between BEE and resting energy expenditure (REE) (RMR extrapolated to 24 hours). BMR is measured under a specific set of circumstances: the subject must be awake, lying comfortably in a supine position, in a state of rest, in a warm room, at least 12 hours after last food ingestion. Since these strict conditions are hard to achieve in hospital settings, energy requirements are usually expressed as RMR. Basal, resting and sleeping energy expenditures are related to body size, being most closely correlated with the size of the fat-free mass (FFM), which is the weight of the body less the weight of its fat mass. The size of the FFM generally explains about 70–80% of the variance in RMR. However, RMR is also affected by age, gender, nutritional state, inherited variations and by differences in the endocrine state, notably (but rarely) by hypo- or hyperthyroidism.

What are the other two components of energy expenditure?

The other two components of energy expenditure are (1) the energy spent on daily activities and physical exercise (which depends on the kind, the intensity and the duration of the physical activity) and (2) the energy spent in response to a variety of thermogenic stimuli (thermogenesis), which include the food we consume, certain drugs, low temperatures, muscle tension, stress and similar psychological states.

What is the thermic effect of food?

It has long been known that food consumption elicits an increase in energy expenditure, a phenomenon known as the 'thermic effect of food' (TEF). The intensity and duration of meal-induced TEF is determined primarily by the amount and composition of the food consumed, mainly owing to the metabolic costs incurred in handling and storing ingested nutrients. Activation of the sympathetic nervous system, elicited by dietary carbohydrate and by sensory stimulation, causes an additional, but modest, increase in energy expenditure. The increments in energy expenditure during digestion above baseline rates, divided by the energy content of the food consumed, vary from 5 to 10% for carbohydrate, 0 to 5% for fat, and 20 to 30% for protein. The high TEF for protein reflects the relatively high metabolic cost involved in processing the amino acids yielded by the absorption of dietary protein, for protein synthesis or for the synthesis of urea and glucose. In general, consumption of the usual mixture of nutrients is generally considered to elicit increases in energy expenditure equivalent to 10% of the food's energy content.

How is energy expressed?

All forms of energy can be converted to heat and all the energy the body uses is lost as heat. For this reason, the energy that is consumed, stored and spent is expressed as its heat equivalent. The first unit of energy employed in nutrition was the calorie [the amount of energy needed to raise the temperature of 1 gram (g) of water from 14.5 to 15.5°C]. In the context of food and nutrition, the kilocalorie (1000 calories) has been traditionally used. However, in the International System of Units, the basic energy unit is the joule (J), which corresponds to the energy used when a mass of 1 kilogram (kg) is moved through 1 m by a force of 1 newton (N). One $J = 0.239$ calories, so that 1 kcal is equal to 4.186 kJ.

Carbohydrates and fibre

What are carbohydrates and how are they classified?

Carbohydrates, the most prevalent organic molecules, are a valuable source of energy in the human diet. It is estimated that in Western countries more than 40% of the energy intake in an average diet comes from carbohydrates. In developing countries, this amount is even higher. Therefore, carbohydrates can be seen as an important fuel for all living beings. As their name denotes, they are synthesised from carbon dioxide and water during plant photosynthesis.

Dietary carbohydrates may be classified by molecular size into (1) sugars, which can be further subdivided into monosaccharides and disaccharides, (2) oligosaccharides, which can be further subdivided into malto-oligosaccharides and other oligosaccharides, and (3) polysaccharides, which can be further subdivided into starch and non-starch polysaccharides.

The commonest monosaccharides are glucose and fructose, which occur in fruit and vegetables. The best-known disaccharides (consisting of two sugar units) are lactose (which is found in milk), sucrose (common sugar) and maltose. Oligosaccharides, containing 3–10 sugar units, are often breakdown products of polysaccharides, which contain more than 10 sugar units. Polysaccharides differ from sugars in that they are non-sweet and less soluble in water. Examples of polysaccharides include starch and glycogen, which are the storage forms of carbohydrates in plants and animals, respectively. Finally, sugar alcohols, such as sorbitol and mannitol, are alcohol forms of glucose and fructose, respectively.

According to an older broad categorisation, carbohydrates may also be classed as (1) simple carbohydrates (known as simple sugars), which are chemically made up of one or two sugar units and are digested quickly, and (2) complex carbohydrates (or starches), which are made of three or more linked sugar units and take longer to absorb. The latter lead to a slower and more stable release of glucose in the blood and are considered healthier.

In the 1920s, according to another categorisation, carbohydrates were divided into (1) available ones (digested and absorbed in the small intestine and providing carbohydrates for metabolism) and (2) unavailable ones (carbohydrates passing to the large intestine and offering substrate for intestinal microflora). The latter were later largely replaced with the term 'dietary fibre', although the two terms are not entirely synonymous.

What are the main functions of carbohydrates?

As mentioned above, carbohydrates have a very crucial role in our diet as an energy source indispensable for the body, and especially for the tissues of the central nervous system, given the fact that the brain has a limited ability to use other energy sources. Carbohydrate energy content is estimated to be 3.75 kcal/g (15.7 kJ/g). Apart from that, they also serve as a structural element in bacteria, plants and animals. Moreover, they help in vitamin and mineral absorption.

Another well-known function of carbohydrates is to impart sweetness to our food. In addition to that, starch, structural polysaccharides and many oligosaccharides have various other roles. For instance, polydextrose adds texture to certain food items. Thanks to their versatility, carbohydrates are widely used in the food industry, for example as thickeners, stabilisers, emulsifiers, crystallisation inhibitors, gelling agents, etc.

What are the minimum and maximum carbohydrate amounts required by humans?

The minimum intake of dietary carbohydrate which is compatible with life can be extremely low, provided that there is an adequate intake of protein and fat amounts, in order to promote *de novo* synthesis of glucose through the hydrolysis of endogenous or dietary protein or glycerol derived from fat. Generally, it is accepted that the minimum carbohydrate amount we need on a daily basis is 100 g [380 kcal (1590 kJ)]. If this minimum requirement is not covered, the result will be the extensive breakdown of body protein, as well as significant salt and water loss.

A diet low in carbohydrates may also lead to bone mineral loss, hyperc-holesterolaemia, and mainly in ketogenesis and ketone-body production in the mitochondria of liver cells. Ketogenesis is the natural response of the body to a low-carbohydrate diet, owing to the exhaustion of cellular carbohydrate stores, such as glycogen and energy production through fatty acids.

For this reason, professional associations such as the British and the American Dietetic Association do not recommend low-carbohydrate diets, which usually are especially high in fat and protein. Low-carbohydrate diets restrict caloric intake by reducing the consumption of carbohydrates to 20–60 g per day (typically less than 20% of the recommended daily caloric intake).

The maximum daily amount of glucose tolerated by an average person is about 400 g. Excessive glucose intake may result in hyperglycaemia. It is generally recognised that the high consumption of sugars – and especially sucrose – has adverse effects on health as it is related to dental caries and chronic diseases, such as diabetes mellitus, obesity, heart disease, etc. Therefore, plasma concentrations of glucose must be carefully regulated.

What is the glycaemic index?

The glycaemic index (GI) is a classification proposed to quantify the relative blood glucose response to foods containing carbohydrate. It is defined as the area under the curve for the increase in blood glucose after the ingestion of a set amount of carbohydrate in an individual food (e.g. 50 g) in the two-hour post-ingestion period as compared with ingestion of the same amount of carbohydrate from a reference food (white bread or glucose) tested in the same individual, under the same conditions, using the initial blood glucose concentration as a baseline. The consumption of foods that have a low GI is beneficial for health as it contributes to good glycaemic control and to the reduction of chronic disease risk factors. Carbohydrates with a high GI cause higher insulin secretion; this is why the GI of dietary carbohydrates, along with the insulinaemic response to them, is of utmost importance for diabetes control.

What is the definition of dietary fibre?

The concept of dietary fibre has changed considerably in recent years. It is now recognised that dietary fibre encompasses a much broader range of substances than was acknowledged previously and that it has greater physiological significance than previously thought. There is no generally accepted definition of dietary fibre worldwide. However, there is a consensus that a physiologically based definition is necessary. The most recent definitions of dietary fibre emanate from the American Association of Cereal Chemists, the US Institute of Medicine, the Agence Française de Sécurité Sanitaire des

Aliments, the Codex Alimentarius Commission and the Health Council of The Netherlands. These definitions all take into account the physiological characteristics of dietary fibre, but with a varying emphasis, and are summarised in Table 1.1.

Early chemistry of non-starch polysaccharides extracted different fibre fractions by controlling the pH of solutions; in this context the terms 'soluble' and 'insoluble' fibre evolved. They provided a useful simple categorisation of dietary fibre with different physiological properties, as understood at the time. Historically, soluble fibres principally affected glucose and fat absorption, because many of them were viscous and formed gels in the small intestine (e.g. pectins and ß-glucans). In contrast, types of dietary fibre with a greater influence on bowel function were referred to as 'insoluble' (including cellulose and lignin). It is now apparent that this simple physiological distinction is inappropriate because some insoluble fibres are rapidly fermented and some soluble fibres do not affect glucose and fat absorption. As the terms 'soluble' and 'insoluble' may be misleading, in 1998 the WHO and the Food and Agricultural Organization recommended that they should no longer be used.

In general, dietary fibres consist primarily of carbohydrate polymers (non-starch polysaccharides) that are components of plant cell walls, including cellulose, hemicellulose and pectins, as well as other polysaccharides of plant or algal origin, such as gums and mucilages and oligosaccharides such as inulin. Analogous non-digestible carbohydrates that pass through the small intestine unchanged but are fermented in the large intestine should also be included, for example resistant starch, fructo-oligosaccharides, galacto-oligosaccharides, modified celluloses and synthesised carbohydrate polymers, such as polydextrose. Associated substances, principally lignin, and minor compounds including waxes, cutin, saponins, polyphenols, phytates and phytosterols, are also included, insofar as they are extracted with the polysaccharides and oligosaccharides in various fibre analytical methods. However, with the exception of lignin, these associated substances when isolated could not be described as dietary fibre. Table 1.2 summarises the most common natural sources of various components of dietary fibre.

In what way is dietary fibre beneficial for health?

Although more studies are certainly needed, it has been suggested that an insufficient consumption of dietary fibre contributes to a plethora of chronic disorders such as constipation, diverticulitis, haemorrhoids, appendicitis, varicose veins, diabetes, obesity, cardiovascular disease, cancer of the large bowel and various other cancers.

What are the recommended fibre intakes through the life cycle?

Recommendations for adult dietary fibre intake generally fall in the range of 20–35 g/day. Others have recommended dietary fibre intakes based on energy intake, 10–13 g of dietary fibre per 1000 kcal. Nutrition fact labels use

Table 1.1 Recent definitions of dietary fibre.

American Association of Cereal Chemists (AACC, 2001)
The edible parts of plants or analogous carbohydrates that are resistant to digestion and absorption in the human small intestine, with complete or partial fermentation in the large intestine. Dietary fibre includes polysaccharides, oligosaccharides, lignin and associated plant substances. Dietary fibres promote beneficial physiological effects, including laxation and/or blood cholesterol attenuation and/or blood glucose attenuation.

Dietary Reference Intakes for Energy, Carbohydrates, Fibre, Fat, Protein and Amino Acids (Macronutrients), Institute of Medicine (2002)
Dietary fibre consists of non-digestible carbohydrates and lignin that are intrinsic and intact in plants.
Functional fibre consists of isolated, non-digestible carbohydrates that have beneficial physiological effects in humans.
Total fibre is the sum of dietary fibre and functional fibre.

Agence Française de Sécurité Sanitaire des Aliments (AFSSA, 2002)
Dietary fibre consists of:
● carbohydrate polymers (degree of polymerisation ≥3) of plant origin with lignin or other non-carbohydrate components (e.g. polyphenols, waxes, saponins, cutin, phytates, phytosterols) AND
● carbohydrate polymers (degree of polymerisation ≥3), processed (by physical, enzymatic or chemical means) or synthetic.

In addition, dietary fibre is neither digested nor absorbed in the small intestine. It has at least one of the following properties:
● stimulates colonic fermentation
● reduces pre-prandial cholesterol levels
● reduces postprandial blood sugar and/or insulin levels.

Codex Alimentarius Commission (CAC, 2006)
Dietary fibre means carbohydrate polymers[a] with a degree of polymerisation not lower than 3, which are neither digested nor absorbed in the small intestine. A degree of polymerisation not lower than 3 is intended to exclude mono- and disaccharides. It is not intended to reflect the average degree of polymerisation of a mixture.
Dietary fibre consists of one or more of:
● edible carbohydrate polymers naturally occurring in the food as consumed
● carbohydrate polymers, which have been obtained from food raw material by physical, enzymatic, or chemical means
● synthetic carbohydrate polymers.
Dietary fibre generally has properties that:
● decrease intestinal transit time and increase stool bulk
● are fermentable by colonic microflora
● reduce blood total and/or low-density lipoprotein cholesterol levels
● reduce postprandial blood glucose and/or insulin levels.

Health Council of the Netherlands (2006)
Dietary fibre is the collective term for substances that are not digested or absorbed in the human small intestine, and which have the chemical structure of carbohydrates, compounds analogous to carbohydrates, and lignin and related substances.

[a] When from plant origin, dietary fibre may include fractions of lignin and/or other compounds when associated with polysaccharides in plant cell walls. Fractions of lignin and/or other compounds (e.g. proteic fractions, phenolic compounds, waxes, saponins, phytates, cutin, phytosterols) intimately associated with plant polysaccharides are included in the definition of fibre insofar as they are actually associated with the poly- or oligosaccharidic fraction of fibre.

Table 1.2 Natural sources of various components of dietary fibre.

Fibre component	Main food source
Cellulose	Vegetables, woody plants, cereal brans
Hemicellulose	Cereal grains
Lignin	Cereal brans, rice and legume hulls, woody plants
Beta-glucans	Grains (oats, barley, rye, wheat)
Pectins	Fruits, vegetables, legumes, sugar beet, potato
Gums	Legumes, seaweed, micro-organisms (guar, locust bean, carrageenan, xanthan, Arabic gum)
Inulin and oligofructose/ fructo-oligosaccharides	Chicory, Jerusalem artichoke, onions
Oligosaccharides	Human milk, grain legumes
Resistance starches:	
Type 1 (RS1)	Starch that is physically inaccessible (e.g. enclosed within intact cell structures in foods such as leguminous seeds and partly milled cereal grains and seeds).
Type 2 (RS2)	Native starch granules (e.g. in maize rich in amylose, raw potatoes, green bananas).

25 g dietary fibre per day for a 2000 kcal/day (8374 kJ/day) diet or 30 g/day for a 2500 kcal/day (10467 kJ/day) diet as goals for American intake. Attempts have been made to define recommended dietary fibre intakes for children and adolescents. Although based on limited clinical data, the recommendation for children older than 2 years is to increase dietary fibre intake to an amount equal to or greater than their age plus 5 g/day and to achieve intakes of 25–35 g/day after age 20 years. No published studies have defined desirable fibre intakes for infants and children younger than 2 years. Until there is more information about the effects of dietary fibre in the very young, a rational approach would be to introduce a variety of fruits, vegetables and easily digested cereals as solid foods are brought into the diet. Specific recommendations for older people have not been published, although a safe recommendation would encourage intakes of 10–13 g dietary fibre per 1000 kcal (4186 kJ). All recommendations need to recognise the importance of adequate fluid intake, and caution should be used when recommending fibre to those with gastrointestinal diseases, including constipation.

Fats and lipids

What are fats and what are lipids?

Lipids form a broad category comprising fats, oils, waxes and various other compounds like lipoproteins, phospholipids and cholesterol. They are all water-insoluble and very useful for living organisms. Fats are food components insoluble in water that represent a condensed source of energy. From a chemical aspect, they are fatty acids, and from a nutritional aspect, they include fatty acids and other lipids, such as phospholipids, sterols, such as cholesterol, and synthetic lipids. One gram of fat provides around 9 kcal (37.7 kJ) of energy.

What are the main functions of fats?

Fats, thanks to their high energy density, are used by the organism as a long-term fuel reserve. Additionally, they act as solvents in the absorption of fat-soluble vitamins and they are the precursors for hormone synthesis, while they also form an integral structural part of cell membranes, in which they play various specific roles (e.g. acting as a pulmonary surfactant, participating in cell signalling, etc.).

In what ways are essential fatty acids important?

Linoleic acid, an omega-6 polyunsaturated fatty acid, and alpha-linolenic acid, an omega-3 polyunsaturated fatty acid, are called 'essential fatty acids' because they are indispensable for our health and they cannot be synthesised by our body, so they have to be obtained through the diet. Linoleic acid is the precursor to arachidonic acid, which is the substrate for eicosanoid production in tissues, is a component of membrane structural lipids and is important in cell signalling pathways. Lack of linoleic acid may lead to various problems, such as skin rash, dermatitis and hair loss. Moreover, lack of alpha-linolenic acid results in adverse clinical symptoms, including neurological abnormalities and poor growth. Clinical and epidemiological studies have addressed the omega-6/omega-3 fatty acid ratio, focusing on the beneficial effects on risk of certain diseases associated with higher intakes of the omega-3 fatty acids eicosapentaenoic acid (EPA) and docosahexaenoic acid (DHA). A linoleic/alpha-linolenic acid ratio of 5:1 to 10:1 has been recommended for adults.

How are dietary fatty acids classified, and which of them are known to be especially beneficial for health?

Dietary fatty acids can be classified into two large categories: saturated (with no double bonds) and unsaturated. The latter are subdivided into monounsaturated fatty acids (MUFA), which have one double bond, and polyunsaturated fatty acids (PUFA), which have more than one double bond. Animal fats tend to be richer in saturated fatty acids compared to vegetable fats.

MUFA are also known as 'omega-9 fatty acids' and the commonest of them is oleic acid. They can be found in olive oil and peanut oil and they are believed to protect against coronary heart disease and some types of cancer. MUFA are a potential fuel source for the body and are critical structural fatty acids for cell membranes and other functions. MUFA are undoubtedly required for many body functions. Nevertheless, MUFA can be biosynthesised from other fuel sources and therefore are not essential in the diet.

PUFA are further divided into the omega-3 family and the omega-6 family, both of which are known to have positive effects on human health. The primary omega-6 PUFA are:

- 18:2 linoleic acid
- 18:3 gamma-linolenic acid
- 20:3 dihomo-gamma-linolenic acid
- 20:4 arachidonic acid
- 22:4 adrenic acid
- 22:5 docosapentaenoic acid.

Sources of omega-6 PUFA are liquid vegetable oils, including soybean oil, corn oil and sunflower oil. Omega-3 PUFA tend to be highly unsaturated with one of the double bonds located at three carbon atoms from the methyl end. This group includes:

- 18:3 alpha-linolenic acid
- 20:5 eicosapentaenoic acid
- 22:5 docosapentaenoic acid
- 22:6 docosahexaenoic acid.

Plant sources of omega-3 PUFA (alpha-linolenic acid) include soybean oil, canola oil, walnuts and flaxseed. Alpha-linolenic acid is the precursor for synthesis of EPA and DHA, which are formed in varying amounts in animal tissues, especially fatty fish (e.g. trout, mackerel, herrings, salmon), but not in plant cells. EPA is the precursor of omega-3 eicosanoids, which have been shown to have beneficial effects in preventing coronary heart disease, arrhythmia and thrombosis, as well as to growth and neural development. Omega-3 fatty acids are considered good both for physical and mental health and to function preventively against heart disease and certain cancers. They also seem to have a beneficial effect on rheumatoid arthritis and atopic dermatitis.

Which fatty acids are considered 'bad' for health?

According to epidemiological and clinical studies, trans fatty acids and to a lesser extent saturated fatty acids (mainly from animal products such as meat and dairy) of the diet are positively associated with coronary heart disease, hypertension and insulin resistance. Dairy fats and meat naturally contain trans fatty acids; however, the majority of dietary trans fatty acids are derived from partially hydrogenated oils. Hydrogenation (a process used to manufacture margarine, for instance) converts PUFA to more saturated fat, thus counteracting the effectiveness of linolenic acid. Bakery foods, shortenings and fried foods, such as potato chips, French fries, etc., are rich in trans fatty acids and their consumption should be avoided.

What are lipoproteins and what is their function in the human body?

Lipoproteins are specialised compounds whose function is to transport through blood circulation lipids to tissues where they are needed. They consist of triacylglycerols and cholesterol esters, phospholipids and free cholesterol, as well as specific proteins, called 'apoproteins', which are important for lipoprotein structure, solubility and metabolism.

Lipoprotein density depends on their lipid/protein ratio. According to the density then, lipoproteins can be divided into four classes: (1) chylomicrons, (2) very low-density lipoproteins (VLDL), (3) low-density lipoproteins (LDL) and high-density lipoproteins (HDL).

Chylomicrons, which are low-density particles formed in the gut, transport dietary lipids to the liver and elsewhere in the body. In the liver, chylomicrons are converted into VLDL, which are the least dense lipoproteins. VLDL and LDL, which are derived from VLDL metabolism, transport fat to the cells. LDL and HDL are responsible for cholesterol transport. LDL transport cholesterol to the cells, while HDL remove excess cholesterol from the cells and carry it back to the liver for breakdown and elimination (reverse cholesterol transport).

A chief dietary goal for arteriosclerotic cardiovascular disease prevention is the reduction of LDL and the increase of HDL. It has been found that a high proportion of individuals who have a myocardial infarction have low HDL.

What is cholesterol and what is its main role in the human body?

Although it is often classified as a lipid, cholesterol belongs in effect to the class of sterols and consists of carbon, hydrogen and oxygen bound in ring structures. It has a vital role as a precursor for the synthesis of bile acids, vitamin D and the steroid hormones, including cortisol, aldosterone and sex hormones. It also has a central role in cell membrane synthesis.

Cholesterol is very susceptible to oxidation. Oxidised cholesterol is involved in the lesions that are responsible for atherosclerosis; therefore, it is implicated in the pathogenesis of heart disease. The main dietary sources of cholesterol are foods of animal origin like eggs, meat and dairy products, as well as certain sea foods, such as lobster, shrimps, etc.

What is the dietary allowance for fat and to what extent should different types of fatty acids be consumed?

Fat provides more calories per gram than any other nutrient [i.e. 9 kcal/g (37.7 kJ/g)] and its addition to food or diet increases their energy density. According to the dietary reference value (DRV) for fat intake, saturated fatty acid (SFA) should provide an average of 10% of total daily energy intake, MUFA (predominately oleic acid) should contribute 12% of total daily energy intake for the population, while the intake for PUFA should not exceed 10%

of total daily energy intake. In particular, the intake of linoleic acid (omega-6 PUFA) should provide 1% of total energy intake and the intake of linolenic acid (omega-3 PUFA) should provide at least 0.2% of total energy intake. Trans fatty acids on the other hand should not exceed 5 g/day or 2% of total daily energy intake. In conclusion, total fatty acid intake should contribute an average of 30% of total energy intake. Total fat intake, calculated by summing up the percentages of SFA, PUFA, MUFA, trans fatty acids and glycerol, should contribute up to 33% of total energy intake including alcohol or 35% of total energy intake derived from food.

According to the *Dietary Guidelines for Americans* produced by the US Department of Health and Human Services, fat intake should not exceed 35%, as higher intakes usually increase the risk of overweight and obesity and should not be less than 20% of total energy intake, as in this case there is a risk of inadequate intakes of essential fatty acids and fat-soluble vitamins and the risk of an adverse effect on high-density lipoprotein cholesterol (HDLC). Therefore, according to the *Guidelines*, total fat intake should be kept between 20 and 35% of total energy intake, mainly from MUFA and PUFA. SFA should not exceed 10% of total energy intake, dietary cholesterol should be limited to 300 mg/day and consumption of trans fatty acids should be as low as possible.

Proteins and amino acids

What are proteins and what are their main functions?

Proteins are the most complex macronutrients and the chemical building blocks composing our body. Their name derives from the Greek term *proteus*, which represents their high importance. They consist of one or more linear chains of amino acids. The size, shape and length of proteins depend on these amino acids and their interactions. In our body, there are 30,000–50,000 different proteins that are broken down and replaced at various rates (protein turnover).

Proteins are essential for life processes, as they are involved in acid–base balance, fluid regulation, immunity, growth, differentiation, gene expression, metabolism and many other functions. They also provide 4 kcal/g (16.7 kJ/g) of energy.

What are the best dietary sources of proteins?

The quality of proteins depends on the essential amino acids they consist of, as well as their digestibility, their absorptive capacity and their biological value. Proteins from animals, such as milk, eggs, meat and fish, are considered to be of higher quality than proteins derived from plant sources (e.g. legumes, grains and vegetables), because the latter lack various essential amino acids. Vegetarian diets are based on the principle of protein complementation, namely the consumption of plant protein sources complementing one another, for instance vegetables and legumes or bread and peanut butter.

What is the current recommended daily protein intake and what factors influence protein requirements?

The currently recommended daily protein intake is 0.8 g/kg (0.37 g/lb) body weight for adult men and women. Protein requirements are influenced by many factors, including growth, the need to replace losses and the need to respond to environmental stimuli.

Protein deficiency seldom occurs independently; more often than not, it occurs along with energy and macronutrient deficiency because of inadequate food intake. Protein energy malnutrition is the commonest type of malnutrition in developing countries. Another condition caused by the insufficient intake of proteins, calories and nutrients is marasmus, the main symptoms of which are muscle-wasting, depletion of fat, reduced growth, abnormal liver enlargement and skin problems. If protein deficiency is serious and lasts too long, it makes patients vulnerable to diseases and may even result in death.

What are amino acids and what are their functions?

Amino acids are the organic compounds that the proteins are made of. There are numerous amino acids, but only twenty of them can be found in proteins in the human body. Amino acids function as substrates for protein and nucleic acid synthesis, and are involved in protein turnover and enzyme activity regulation, nitrogen transport, oxidation-reduction reaction, etc.

How are amino acids classified?

Amino acids can be classified into essential, non-essential and conditionally essential amino acids. According to another nutritional classification amino acids are categorised into two groups: indispensable (essential) and dispensable (non-essential). The nine indispensable amino acids (Table 1.3) are those that have carbon skeletons that cannot be synthesised to meet the body's needs from simpler molecules in animals, and therefore must be provided in the diet. Dispensable amino acids can be further divided into two classes: truly dispensable and conditionally indispensable. Five of the amino acids are termed dispensable as they can be synthesised in the body from either other amino acids or other complex nitrogenous metabolites. In addition, six other amino acids, including cysteine and tyrosine, are conditionally indispensable as they are synthesised from other amino acids or their synthesis is limited under special pathophysiological conditions. This is even more of an issue in the neonate, where it has been suggested that only alanine, aspartate,

Table 1.3 Indispensable, dispensable and conditionally indispensable amino acids in the human diet.

Indispensable	Dispensable	Conditionally indispensable[a]	Precursors of conditionally indispensable
Histidine[b]	Alanine	Arginine	Glutamine/glutamate,
Isoleucine	Aspartic acid	Cysteine	aspartate
Leucine	Asparagine	Glutamine	Methionine, serine
Lysine	Glutamic acid	Glycine	Glutamic acid/ammonia
Methionine	Serine	Proline	Serine, choline
Phenylalanine		Tyrosine	Glutamate
Threonine			Phenylalanine
Tryptophan			
Valine			

[a] Conditionally indispensable is defined as requiring a dietary source when endogenous synthesis cannot meet metabolic need.
[b] Although histidine is considered indispensable, unlike the other eight indispensable amino acids, it does not fulfil the criteria used in this report of reducing protein deposition and inducing negative nitrogen balance promptly upon removal from the diet.
Source: Laidlaw SA, Kopple JD (1987) Newer concepts of the indispensable amino acids. *American Journal of Clinical Nutrition.* **46**(4): 593–605.

glutamate, serine and probably asparagine are truly dispensable. The term 'conditionally indispensable' recognises the fact that under most normal conditions the body can synthesise these amino acids to meet metabolic needs. However, there may be certain physiological circumstances: prematurity in the young infant, where there is an inadequate rate at which cysteine can be produced from methionine; the newborn, where enzymes that are involved in quite complex synthetic pathways may be present in inadequate amounts, as in the case of arginine, which results in a dietary requirement for this amino acid; or pathological states, such as severe catabolic stress in an adult, where the limited tissue capacity to produce glutamine to meet increased needs and to balance increased catabolic rates makes a dietary source of these amino acids required to achieve body nitrogen homeostasis. The small intestine's cells become important sites of the synthesis of conditionally indispensable amino acid and hence some amino acids (e.g. glutamine and arginine) become nutritionally indispensable under circumstances of intestinal metabolic dysfunction. However, the quantitative requirement levels for conditionally indispensable amino acids have not been determined and these, presumably, vary greatly according to the specific condition.

Amino acids can also be classified according to their structure into aromatic amino acids, which are precursors of neurotransmitters such as dopamine, epinephrine and serotonin, and branched-chain amino acids, which are selectively taken up by muscle cells rather than the liver. The former include phenylalanine, tryptophan and occasionally histidine, while the latter include isoleucine, leucine and valine.

Vitamins

What are vitamins and how are they classified?

Vitamins are micronutrients necessary for the maintenance of normal metabolic functions and blood cell formation. They are not synthesised in adequate amounts in the human body, so they have to be obtained through the diet, as vitamin deficiencies may lead to various dysfunctions.

Vitamins include 13 different organic molecules, which, despite their structural and functional heterogeneity, may be classified into two main categories, as seen in Table 1.4.

Water-soluble vitamins are rapidly depleted and must be regularly replenished, while fat-soluble (lipid-soluble) vitamins are better stored in the body. Vitamins can also be divided into natural and synthetic ones. Their action and kinetics are similar.

Can vitamins become harmful to health?

Many vitamins can have serious side effects or even prove to be toxic if taken in excess; this is why megadoses must be avoided. This applies especially to the fat-soluble vitamins, as they can accumulate in the body, reaching potentially dangerous levels.

Vitamin A and D toxicity syndromes are well documented, while vitamin K may also be toxic in water-soluble form. Some examples of well-known side effects due to vitamin excess are:

- headaches (vitamin A)
- vomiting (vitamins A and D)
- nausea (vitamins D, C, nicotinamide, vitamin B_6)
- spontaneous abortions and birth defects (vitamin A)
- diarrhoea (vitamin C, pantothenic acid, choline, carnitine)
- haemolytic anaemia and kernicterus (vitamin K)
- hepatomegaly (vitamin A, niacin).

Table 1.4 Vitamin classifications.

Water-soluble vitamins	Fat-soluble vitamins
B-complex vitamins	
Thiamin (B_1)	Vitamin A
Riboflavin (B_2)	Vitamin D
Niacin (B_3)	Vitamin E
Pantothenic acid (B_5)	Vitamin K
Pyridoxine (B_6)	
Biotin	
Cobalamin (B_{12})	
Folic acid	
Ascorbic acid (C)	

Which groups of people are at greatest risk of vitamin deficiency?

Although it is preferable to follow a balanced diet that covers all the vitamin needs of the body, vitamin supplements are sometimes indicated for groups of people that may be at risk of developing certain deficiencies. Eligible candidates for vitamin supplementation may be:

- the very young, and especially premature infants
- pregnant women
- the very old
- some categories of people suffering from chronic diseases, and especially chronically undernourished patients and chronic alcoholics, who commonly develop thiamin deficiency
- injured people, given the fact that vitamins (and especially ascorbic acid) play a role in wound healing
- strict vegetarians (vegans), who may be at increased risk of developing specific vitamin deficiencies.

The importance of vitamins for health is widely publicised today, and certain vitamins (beta-carotene, vitamin E and vitamin C) are believed to be involved in the prevention of oxidative damage caused by free radicals; therefore, they have been linked to the potential prevention of cancer, atherosclerosis and heart disease. For this reason, many people, especially in Western societies, choose to supplement their diets with vitamins that they strongly believe are good for their health. It must be stressed, however, that since the antioxidant action of the above mentioned vitamins has not been fully elucidated yet and more studies are evidently needed, vitamin supplements ideally should be taken on prescription and only after careful evaluation of each individual's nutritional status. In addition, patients should be warned of the dangers of the excessive intake of vitamins, and especially vitamins A, D, E and K.

Which foods are good sources of vitamin?

Most water-soluble vitamins are generally found in the same groups of foods, namely whole grains, leafy vegetables, legumes, meat and dairy products.

Food sources of vitamin C (ascorbic acid) are fresh fruit (and especially citrus fruit) and vegetables. Vitamin B_{12} is synthesised by micro-organisms and then becomes incorporated in animal tissues. This is why vegans, who avoid animal products altogether, are at risk of developing B_{12} deficiency.

As for the food sources of fat-soluble vitamins, they generally include leafy vegetables, seed oils, meat and full-fat dairy products.

More specifically, as far as vitamin A is concerned, it should be noted that the term includes both retinol and provitamin A carotenoids. Liver, fortified margarine and full-fat milk products are good dietary sources of retinol and bright orange fruits and vegetables (e.g. carrots, pumpkins, sweet potatoes, apricots) and dark-green vegetables (e.g. peppers, spinach, broccoli) are the best sources of carotenes.

The dietary sources of vitamin D, which are not as important as its endogenous synthesis on the skin by the sunlight, however, are oily fish, eggs, liver, full-fat dairy products and fortified milk.

Oily fish and green leafy vegetables are also rich in vitamin E. Other good sources of vitamin E are seeds, vegetable oils and beans.

The main food sources of vitamin K are nuts and seeds, as well as nut oils and seed oils.

Minerals and trace elements

What are minerals and trace elements?

Minerals and trace elements are required in only small or even trace quantities, but are nonetheless essential for normal bodily function. They exhibit a variety of roles and are often necessary for tissue structure, enzyme system function, fluid balance, cellular function and neurotransmission. The elements that are required in milligram quantities (sometimes several hundred milligrams) are called 'minerals'; those required in microgram quantities are known as 'trace elements'. Table 1.5 summarises the minerals and trace elements that are known to be essential for humans and Table 1.6 presents the reference nutrient intakes (RNIs) for adults, for some selected minerals and trace elements.

What role does calcium play in human health?

Calcium is the most abundant inorganic chemical in the human body – it accounts for 1.5–2% of our body weight – and is the main mineral of bones and teeth (approximately 90% of the calcium present in the human body can be found in bones and teeth). Bone calcium content changes with age, body size and body composition. Calcium is necessary for the regulation of neural

Table 1.5 Trace elements present in the human body.

Essential	Potentially essential
Chromium (Cr)	Aluminium (Al)
Cobalt (Co)	Arsenic (As)
Copper (Cu)	Boron (B)
Fluoride (F)	Cadmium (Cd)
Iodine (I)	Nickel (Ni)
Iron (Fe)	Silicon (Si)
Manganese (Mn)	Vanadium (V)
Molybdenum (Mo)	
Selenium (Se)	
Zinc (Zn)	

Table 1.6 Mineral RNIs for adults.

Age	Calcium mg/d	Phosphorus mg/d	Magnesium mg/d	Sodium mg/d	Potassium mg/d	Chloride mg/d	Iron mg/d	Copper mg/d	Selenium μg/d	Iodine μg/d
Males										
19–50 years	700	550	300	1600	3500	2500	8.7	1.2	75	140
50+ years	700	550	300	1600	3500	2500	8.7	1.2	75	140
Females										
19–50 years	700	550	270	1600	3500	2500	14.8	1.2	60	140
50+ years	700	550	270	1600	3500	2500	8.7	1.2	60	140

Chapter 1

and muscular functions, the good hormonal functioning of the body, normal blood coagulation, effective digestion, etc.

The RNI for calcium is 400–1200 mg. Women's needs are higher than men's are, especially during lactation. Calcium supplements may be needed for the prevention of osteoporosis, a condition especially prevalent among older women.

Foods rich in calcium are milk and dairy products, cruciferous vegetables (e.g. broccoli, cauliflower, Brussels sprouts), mineral waters, almonds and legumes.

What is the role of phosphorus in the human body?

Phosphorus is the second most abundant inorganic compound in the body after calcium. Most of the total phosphorus present in our body can be found in the bones, along with calcium. Phosphorus also plays an important role in carbohydrate, lipid and protein metabolism.

The RNI for phosphorus intake is 550 mg. Phosphorus-rich food sources are milk, meat, poultry, fish, nuts and cereals.

How important is sodium for our health?

Sodium, along with potassium and chloride, is involved in body fluid osmolarity and plays the most decisive role in determining extracellular osmolarity. It is necessary for the good functioning of the nervous system and the muscles.

Our daily physiological requirements are small and equal to 69–460 mg/day, while the RNI for sodium for adults is 1600 mg/day (70 mmol/d) (6 g/day of salt or 2.4 g/day of sodium). These requirements can be covered from the foods we consume, without the addition of extra salt (sodium chloride), which has been associated with hypertension, renal problems, etc.

Why is iron essential?

Iron has multiple biochemical roles in the human body. It is necessary for the production of red blood cells and haemoglobin. As the major component of haemoglobin, it is necessary for the transport of oxygen to cells throughout the body. Iron also reinforces the defensive mechanisms of the body against illnesses.

The depletion of the body's iron stores leads to disorders. The most important of these is iron-deficiency anaemia, which is the commonest nutritional deficiency syndrome in the world. Consequently, our diet must contain adequate amounts of iron-containing foods, such as liver, meat, poultry, shellfish, eggs, fish, apricots, lentils, beans, etc. The RNI for men is 8.7 mg daily, while for women it is 14.8 mg daily. Daily requirements are higher during the early developmental stages, pregnancy and lactation.

It must be noted, however, that excess iron, which can be accumulated under certain conditions, is harmful as well, as it can be toxic to cells and tissues. Two pathological conditions associated with iron overload are haemosiderosis, in which too much iron is deposited in the tissues, and haemochromatosis, a rather rare, genetically predetermined disease.

Why do we need zinc and what are our daily requirements?

Zinc is necessary for a broad range of biochemical processes that are important for growth and development and zinc deficiency results in poor healing and growth retardation. The RNI for zinc is 9.5 mg for men and 7.0 mg for women daily. Its best dietary sources are whole grains, nuts, meat, fish and poultry.

What is iodine useful for?

Iodine is considered essential because it is a constituent of hormones thyroxin and triiodothyronine, which are necessary for normal physical and mental growth (i.e. maintenance of metabolic rate, thermoregulation, protein synthesis, connective tissue integrity). Its best dietary source is fish and seafood. The RNI for iodine is 140 μg daily, with no increment during lactation and pregnancy.

What is the role of chromium?

Chromium has been considered an essential trace element for the last two decades, since it was found that it is important for glucose regulation. It seems that as an insulin cofactor it contributes to insulin binding to the cell membrane, while it is also involved in maintaining normal blood glucose levels and in triglyceride level regulation. The estimated safe and adequate daily intake of chromium is 120 μg or 0.5 μmol/day for adults and 0.1 and 1.0 μg/kg/day (2 and 19 nmol/kg/day) for children and adolescents respectively. Doses larger than 200 μg are toxic and may cause concentration problems and fainting. The best chromium food sources are yeast, liver, potatoes, bran, seafood, meat and poultry.

Is fluoride essential?

Fluoride is valuable for healthy bones and teeth and it has been shown to prevent dental caries. There is little evidence that there is any physiological requirement for fluoride and therefore no RNIs have been set; however, it has been suggested that the continuous fluoridation of water supplies to achieve levels of 1 ppm (parts per million) is generally recommended. Water, therefore, is the best source of fluoride, although its content may vary from one area to another. Fluoride is also found in several foods, which provide about 25% of total intake. Fluoride is considered as semi-essential since, although no physiological requirement can be shown to exist, it has known beneficial effects.

Food models

What are the food models and which are the most widely used?

Food guide models are mainly teaching instruments that can be used in order to educate the general population on healthy eating and to visualise the frequency of consumption of the different food groups. They are most frequently in the form of a pyramid or a plate and are divided into sections, according to the number of food groups (e.g. fruits, cereals, fats, vegetables). The size of every section represents the frequency of food or food group consumption; although in some of the food models there are certain numeric suggestions for food consumption and for portions. In some of these models, there are suggestions for exercise, fluid consumption and alcohol.

What is the Food Guide Pyramid and how can it be used?

The Food Guide Pyramid is a practical graphic developed by the US Department of Agriculture (USDA) in 1992. It was designed to serve as a teaching instrument to offer guidance to the public concerning food choice and portion size. It divides foods into five main groups and gives the number of recommended servings for each. It is organised to facilitate the interpretation of the given information by non-experts: at the base of the pyramid we can find foods that are considered to form the basis of the diet and as we move upwards we come across groups of foods that we should consume less of, until we reach the pyramid top, where we can find foods to be used only sparingly (Table 1.7). The Food Guide Pyramid has not been revised so far, so it is officially still valid, although it no longer agrees with the *Dietary Guidelines for Americans* (Figure 1.1), which have changed already twice since the creation of the pyramid.

Concerns have been raised about the base of the pyramid, which recommends too many carbohydrates without any reference to the differences between good (complex) carbohydrates versus refined ones and sugars. In view of new scientific data, many experts also criticise the pyramid's message to avoid fat.

What is the Balance of Good Health plate?

The Balance of Good Health plate was the food model suggested and most widely used in UK, which showed the types and proportions of foods needed

Table 1.7 The Food Guide Pyramid: the main sections, the food groups and the suggested servings of the pyramid.

Fats, Oils and Sweets Use sparingly **Milk, Yogurt and Cheese Group** 2–3 servings **Meat, Poultry, Fish, Dry Beans, Eggs and Nuts Group** 2–3 servings	**Vegetable Group** 3–5 servings **Fruit Group** 2–4 servings **Bread, Cereal, Rice and Pasta Group** 6–11 servings

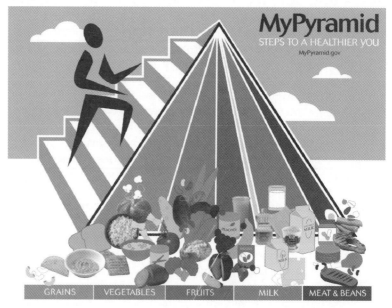

Figure 1.1 The Food Guide Pyramid. (*Source*: United States Department of Agriculture.)

for the balanced diet in a plate, in order to be more comprehensible. The Balance of Good Health plate (Figure 1.2) or the Eatwell Plate (Figure 1.3), which consists of the most recently revised version of the original Balance of Good Health plate, still represent a more pictorial way to express, in a more practical mode, the dietary recommendations for a healthy diet, for the general population.

Are there any other food models available?

There are numerous other pyramids, such as the Mediterranean Diet Pyramid (Figure 1.4), the Soul Food Pyramid, the vegetarian pyramid and many ethnic ones. A pyramid that does not limit guidance only to food choices and quantities is Willett's Healthy Eating Pyramid, a pyramid that gives emphasis

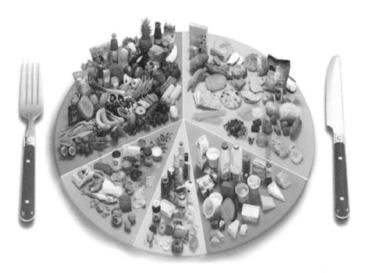

Figure 1.2 The Balance of Good Health plate. © Crown Copyright

to daily physical exercise and weight control, along with abundant consumption of whole grains, vegetables and plant oils. Most of these healthy diet models advise consuming plenty of fruit and vegetables and cutting down on sugar products and refined carbohydrates.

People should generally be encouraged to eat a balanced diet consisting of reasonable choices of all macronutrients, including fats and healthy

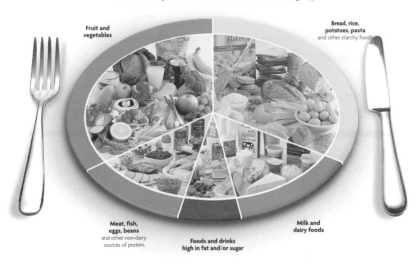

Figure 1.3 The Eatwell Plate. © Crown Copyright

Chapter 1

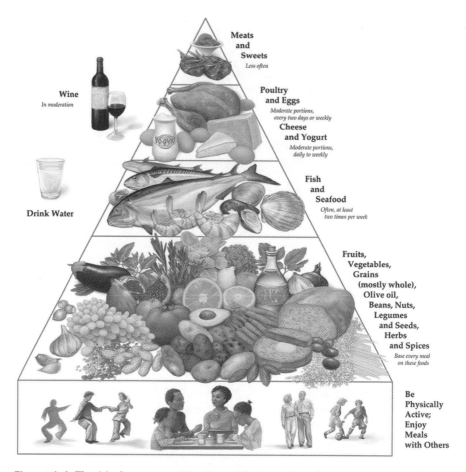

Figure 1.4 The Mediterranean Diet Pyramid. Reproduced with permission. © 2009 Oldways Preservation & Exchange Trust (www.oldwayspt.org). Illustration by George Middleton.

carbohydrates, to maintain a normal body weight and to make physical activity an integral part of their everyday life.

Further reading

American Association of Cereal Chemists (AACC), Dietary Fiber Technical Committee (2001) The definition of dietary fiber. *Cereals Food World* **46**: 112–26.

Atkinson J, Epand RF, Epand RM (2007) Tocopherols and tocotrienols in membranes: A critical review. *Free Radical Biology & Medicine* **44**(5): 739–64.

Chiuve SE, Willett WC (2007) The 2005 Food Guide Pyramid: An opportunity lost? *Nature Clinical Practice Cardiovascular Medicine* **4**(11): 610–20.

Department of Health (1991) *Dietary reference values for food energy and nutrients for the United Kingdom.* Report on Health and Social Subjects, 41. Committee on Medical Aspects of Food Policy. HMSO, London.

EEC Scientific Committee for Food (1993) *Thirty-first Series: Nutrient and energy intakes for the European Community*. Directorate-General, Industry, Luxemburg.

Food and Agriculture Organization/World Health Organization (1997) *Energy and Protein Requirements*. Report of a joint FAO/WHO ad hoc Expert Committee. FAO, Rome.

Food and Agriculture Organization/World Health Organization (1998) *Carbohydrates in Human Nutrition*. Report of a joint FAO/WHO Consultation. FAO Food and Nutrition Paper 66. FAO, Rome.

Gray J (2006) *Dietary Fibre: Definition, analysis, physiology and health*. ILSI Europe, Brussels.

Institute of Medicine (1997) *Dietary Reference Intakes for Calcium, Phosphorus, Magnesium, Vitamin D, and Fluoride*. Food and Nutrition Board. National Academy Press, Washington.

Institute of Medicine (1999) *Dietary Reference Intakes for Thiamin, Riboflavin, Niacin, Vitamin B_6, Folate, Vitamin B_{12}, Pantothenic Acid, Biotin and Choline*. National Academy Press, Washington.

Institute of Medicine (2000) *Dietary Reference Intakes for Vitamin C, Vitamin E, Selenium, and Carotenoids*. Food and Nutrition Board. National Academy Press, Washington.

Institute of Medicine (2001) *Dietary Reference Intakes for Vitamin A, Vitamin K, Arsenic, Boron, Chromium, Copper, Iodine, Iron, Molybdenum, Nickel, Silicon, Vanadium and Zinc*. Food and Nutrition Board. National Academy Press, Washington.

Institute of Medicine (2002) *Dietary Reference Intakes: Energy, Carbohydrate, Fiber, Fat, Fatty Acids, Cholesterol, Protein, and Amino Acids*. National Academy Press, Washington.

Laidlaw SA, Kopple JD (1987) Newer concepts of the indispensable amino acids. *American Journal of Clinical Nutrition* **46**(4): 593–605.

Lanou AJ, Berkow SE, Barnard ND (2005) Calcium, dairy products, and bone health in children and young adults: A re-evaluation of the evidence. *Pediatrics* **115**: 736–43.

Marshall TA (2006) Translating the new dietary guidelines. *Journal of the American Dental Association* **137**(9): 1258–60.

Ministry of Agriculture, Fisheries and Food (1997) *National Food Survey*. The Stationery Office, London.

Ministry of Agriculture, Fisheries and Food (1998) *Fatty Acids: Seventh supplement to the composition of foods*, 5th edn. Royal Society of Chemistry/MAFF, Cambridge.

National Research Council, Food and Nutrition Board, Commission on Life Sciences (1989) *Recommended Dietary Allowances*, 10th edn. National Academy Press, Washington.

Oldways Preservation & Exchange Trust, Boston, MA (www.oldwayspt.org).

Park Y, Hunter DJ, Spiegelman D et al. (2005) Dietary fiber intake and risk of colorectal cancer: A pooled analysis of prospective cohort studies. *Journal of the American Medical Association* **14, 294**(22): 2849–57.

Rolls BJ, Bell EA (1999) Intake of fat and carbohydrate: Role of energy density. *European Journal of Clinical Nutrition* **53**(suppl. 1): S166–73.

Sadovsky R, Collins N, Tighe AP et al. (2008) Dispelling the myths about omega-3 fatty acids. *Postgraduate Medicine* **120**(2): 92–100.

Skulas-Ray AC, West SG, Davidson MH, Kris-Etherton PM (2008) Omega-3 fatty acid concentrates in the treatment of moderate hypertriglyceridemia. *Expert Opinion on Pharmacotherapy* **9**(7): 1237–48.

Chapter 1

Straub DA (2007) Calcium supplementation in clinical practice: A review of forms, doses, and indications. *Nutrition in Clinical Practice* **22**(3): 286.

US Department of Health and Human Services/US Department of Agriculture (2005) *Dietary Guidelines for Americans.* USDHHS/USDA, Washington.

Venn BJ, Green TJ (2007) Glycemic index and glycemic load: Measurement issues and their effect on diet–disease relationships. *European Journal of Clinical Nutrition* **61**(suppl. 1): S122–31.

Wheeler ML, Pi-Sunyer FX (2008) Carbohydrate issues: Type and amount. *Journal of the American Dietetic Association* **108**(4, suppl. 1): S34–9.

Willett WC, Sacks F, Trichopoulou A *et al.* (1995) Mediterranean diet pyramid: A cultural model for healthy eating. *American Journal of Clinical Nutrition* **61**(6, suppl.): S1402–6.

Chapter 2

Nutritional Assessment

Charilaos Dimosthenopoulos

What is nutritional assessment and how can it be completed?

Nutritional assessment is an extremely useful tool for the application of nutritional therapy. It is related to the individual's (1) food and nutrient intake (diet history), (2) lifestyle, (3) medication intake, (4) social and medical history and (5) anthropometric, body composition and biochemical measurements. It includes both the screening and assessment of the person's nutritional status, the collection of data through the use of interviews, questionnaires and specially designed forms and the scientific analysis of the information obtained. These data are used in order to identify the nutritional status of the individual, to design the appropriate nutritional therapy and to investigate the need for greater nutritional support.

What information should be collected from a dietary history?

Taking a dietary history is a common method of evaluating food intake, and was devised by Burke in 1947. It can be made by taking, through an interview, an informative dietary history of an individual or a group of people. This dietary history should provide all the data needed in order to evaluate the food and fluid intake. It consists of a 24-hour recall, a food frequency questionnaire and a three-day food record. Some of the most frequent and necessary information collected is: the usual dietary and meal plan, the number of meals, the usual meal size and the common amount of food, the usual location of eating, the consumption of ready-made meals, snacks and fast food, fluid intake, including the consumption of beverages and alcohol, possible food allergies, food preferences and the frequency of consumption.

What are the strengths and the limitations of the dietary history?

A dietary history can give the dietitian an accurate picture not only of a person's normal food intake but also of the quality of that diet. However, the interview is a time-consuming process requiring well-educated interviewers being able to collaborate successfully with interviewees in order both to generate accurate data about a person's usual dietary intake and to be able to differentiate between the number and content of daily meals (daily meal plan).

What are the advantages and disadvantages of the 24-hour recall method?

The 24-hour recall is a simple method of direct nutritional assessment, which was first used by Wiehl in 1942. Using this method, it is easy to obtain the necessary information concerning the individual's total food and fluid intake, for the previous day or previous 24 hours. It is a quantitative method and is based on the assumption that the intake described is typical of the daily food and drink intake of the individual. The advantages of this method are that it is easy, quick, to a large extent representative and does not need special equipment (e.g. scales). It does not need literacy and is less likely to alter eating behaviour, with a relatively minimal respondent burden. The main disadvantages of this method are: (1) it is dependent on the memory of the individual and thus it is not advisable for individuals with decreased memory skills (older people and young children); (2) it is does not provide accurate information when there is a day-to-day variation of the food intake; and (3) there is usually the tendency from the interviewees asked to declare incorrect food intake (either lower or higher than actual food intake), which may lead to statistical mistakes and unreal results (overestimation appears to be more frequent than underestimation for portion sizes). The role of a well-skilled dietitian or any other health professional involved in this method is essential in order to obtain the data accurately.

How do we select the appropriate method?

The selection of the appropriate method depends on the type of information to be collected. As there is no ideal method that could be used in all the cases and evaluations, each method addresses a different target group (e.g. different age, gender, social, educational group) or a different food or nutrient intake assessment. For the estimation of the actual nutrient intake of individuals or small groups of people for a certain period, food diaries or 24-hour recall are used. For the estimation of the mean dietary and nutrient intake in a large population, repeated 24-hour recalls or food diaries are used, while in the case of the estimation of the mean intake of a certain food item (e.g. specific type of fat, sweetener, fibre), by a small or larger population, a

Table 2.1 Classification of weight status by body mass index.

Classification	BMI (kg/m²)
Underweight	<18.5
Normal weight	18.5–24.9
Overweight	25–29.9
Obesity Class 1	30–34.9
Obesity Class 2	35–39.9
Extreme Obesity Class 3	>40

food frequency questionnaire is used instead. Finally, in the case of the evaluation of a population being in nutritional danger, repeated 24-hour recalls or a food frequency questionnaire are more commonly used.

How can we calculate the body mass index and how should we use it? Is it always reliable?

BMI is the most recommended classification of body weight and one of the simplest and most widely used methods for the estimation of body fat. Developed by the Belgian statistician Adolphe Quetelet, it can be calculated by a simple equation, dividing the subject's weight by the square of his/her height. BMI is typically expressed in either metric or imperial units and constitutes an indicator of the stores of body fat, being related to an increased danger of illness and mortality, for individuals. BMI classifies individuals as underweight, normal weight, overweight or obese. (See Table 2.1 and Table 2.2.)

$$BMI = \frac{Weight\,(in\,kg)}{Height\,(in\,m^2)}$$

Table 2.2 Classification of risk of diabetes (type 2), hypertension and cardiovascular disease associated with body weight.

Classification of overweight and obesity by BMI and waist circumference	Increased risk for obesity-related health problems, e.g. type 2 diabetes, hypertension and cardiovascular disease	
	Waist circumference Women <88 cm Men <102 cm	Waist circumference Women >88 cm Men >102 cm
Underweight (BMI <18.5)		
Normal (BMI 18.5–24.9)		Eventually high (thin obese)
Overweight (BMI 25–29.9)	Increased	High
Obese Class I (BMI 30–34.9)	High	Very high
Obese Class II (BMI 35–39.9)	Very high	Very high
Extreme Obesity Class 3 (BMI >40)	Extremely high	Extremely high

It can be also calculated in US/Customary units: BMI = lb × 703 / in.², where 'lb' is the subject's weight in pounds and 'in.' is the subject's height in inches.

Values of BMI lower than 25 are considered of normal weight. Individuals with BMI of 25–30 are considered overweight, while values over 30 present obesity. Persons with a BMI <18.5 have an increased mortality rate. It should be mentioned, though, that BMI is not directly correlated with the accumulation of body fat, and for this reason there are exceptions (e.g. athletes, who have a very limited level of body fat and cannot be classified as overweight or obese like other adults).

Which anthropometric measurements are the most useful?

The term 'anthropometric' refers to comparative measurements of the body, which are used in nutritional assessments in order to understand human physical variation. The most useful measurements for infants, children and adolescents, which are used to assess growth and development, usually include:

- length
- height
- weight
- weight-for-length
- head circumference (length is used in infants and toddlers, rather than height, because they are unable to stand).

The anthropometric measurements which are used for adults usually include:

- height
- weight
- BMI
- waist/hip ratio
- percentage of body fat.

Is the waist/hip ratio a useful tool for nutritional assessment?

The measurement of circumferences of the human body, for example the area of waist and hip, can be used in order to estimate the distribution of body fat and the danger of the development of certain diseases related to the central distribution of fat. The waist/hip ratio (WHR) is the ratio of the circumference of the waist to that of the hips and is calculated by measuring the waist circumference, just above the upper hip bone and dividing by the hip circumference at its widest part. In several, but not all observational studies, indexes of abdominal adiposity, such as the WHR and waist circumference (WC), predict coronary heart disease and strokes better than BMI, while an increased WHR is related with increased risk of stroke in women.

What are the highest healthy levels of the waist/hip ratio for men and women?

A WHR of 0.7 for women and 0.9 for men has been shown to correlate strongly with a general status of healthy, while values of WHR over 1.0 for men and over 0.8 for women are indicative of the presence of central obesity and increased risk of related diseases (associated with higher risk of diabetes and hypertension). WHRs above 0.95 for men or 0.8 for women indicate a heightened risk of heart attack (Table 2.2).

Is the measurement of wrist circumference a valuable measurement?

Wrist circumference is one of the measurements that have been proposed for the estimation of the size of the frame, which include the width of wrist and knee and are considered valuable. However, the quotient of the height to the wrist circumference and the measurement of width of elbow are two of the more often used measurements of the frame's size. The size of the frame (r) is measured through the following quotient:

$$r = \frac{\text{height (cm)}}{\text{wrist circumference (cm)}}$$

The classification of the frame's size according to the guidelines of the American Dietetic Association is given in Table 2.3.

Which biochemical markers are useful for nutritional evaluation?

Many different biochemical markers can reveal nutritional depletion and play an essential role in nutritional evaluation. As far as concerns the evaluation of vitamins and minerals levels in the body, this can be realised by the measurement of these or their products of metabolism, in the blood, the urine and other biological materials. Serum proteins seem to be useful markers of nutritional status.

Table 2.3 Classification of the size of the frame.

Frame's size	Men	Women
Small	>10.4	>11
Medium	9.6–10.4	10.1–11.0
Large	<9.6	<0.1

Source: Chicago Dietetic Association, The South Shore Suburban Dietetic Association and Dieticians of Canada (2000) Manual of Clinical Dietetics. American Dietetic Association, Chicago, IL.

Serum albumin

The serum albumin level is an indicative marker, for the nutritional evaluation of a patient, although it has a relatively long half-life of 21 days. Patients with low serum albumin levels are in poor nutritional condition and at high risk of death.

Prealbumin

Malnourished patients, according to Subjective Global Assessment – a method of assessing nutritional status – have significantly lower levels of prealbumin. Thus, determining the levels of prealbumin can be a sensitive and cost-effective method of assessing the severity of illness, which can result from malnutrition in patients who are critically ill or have a chronic disease and may allow for earlier recognition and intervention for malnutrition.

Serum creatinine

This protein is used as a nutritional marker, because of its relation to muscle mass. Measuring serum creatinine is a simple test and it is the most commonly used indicator of renal function.

Serum transferrin

This is an iron-transport protein, which serves as a sensitive marker of total nutrition status and more specifically as a marker of iron deficiency. Serum transferrin receptor (sTfR) level is a new specific and sensitive indicator of tissue iron status and iron deficiency.

How can special nutritional requirements be identified?

Nutritional requirements are determined by a wide variety of factors. In order to identify special nutritional requirements and determine the extent to which the individual's nutritional needs are covered, specific parameters and methods are used, which can provide all of the necessary data. The nutritional requirements assessment includes:

- clinical assessment
- physical assessment
- biochemical/haematological assessment
- anthropometric and body composition assessment
- current dietary assessment.

Many specialised methods are generally used by clinical dietitians for this purpose. Subjective Global Assessment (SGA) is one of the most popular and effective methods for the assessment of nutritional status and special nutritional needs. SGA classification is a comprehensive assessment technique and a valid screening tool for the prevention and treatment of, especially, malnutrition or undernutrition, in various patient populations.

How can we estimate protein requirements?

Protein is one of the main macronutrients that are essential for life and growth and vital for the structure and the metabolism of the human body. It is continuously broken down and synthesised (the homeostatic mechanism generally known as protein turnover), but it cannot be stored and thus there is a daily minimum requirement intake to maintain the body's structure and function throughout life. In adults and on a daily basis, approximately 200–300 g of protein or 3–4 g protein/kg body weight is turned over. Protein contains nitrogen and the daily protein requirements are related to the total amount needed to maintain nitrogen equilibrium and cover losses. A general estimation of the protein requirements is based on the current RNIs and RDAs for protein, which are, for the average adult, 0.75–0.8 g/kg of body weight per day, while a more accurate estimation can be made by measuring the nitrogen excretion and total losses (via urine, faeces, fistulae or other losses).

How can we estimate carbohydrate requirements?

Carbohydrate is the main fuel for the human body and the most important dietary energy source, providing approximately 3.8 kcal/g. The total carbohydrate requirements are usually expressed as a percentage (e.g. 45–60% for adults) of the total energy intake, according to the dietary reference values (DRVs) for the main nutrients, from which 39% should derive from starches, milk sugars and intrinsic sugars and not more than 11% from non-milk extrinsic sugars. At the same time, there are general recommendations for carbohydrate intake, in grams. Thus, the minimum daily recommendation for carbohydrate is 100 g, in order to provide enough energy and avoid protein breakdown, and the maximum intake is approximately 400 g for the average adult.

How can we estimate fluid requirements?

Fluid requirements vary considerably between individuals and are influenced by various factors, related to the individual's age, gender, level of physical activity, type of diet, the environmental temperature and the climate, the individual's total fluid intake (from foods, water and beverages) and fluid output (kidney losses, respiratory, skin and gastrointestinal losses) and the general state of the individual's health. Individuals should take no less than the amount of fluids that cover the total losses and no more than the amount that can be excreted by the kidney function. It is recommended that the fluid intake should be at least 500–750 ml greater than urinary losses, but it should be even greater in cases of high temperatures or the presence of burn or pyrexia or in the case of any other reason of higher-than-normal losses.

Chapter 2

Generally and under normal circumstances, the fluid requirements can be estimated:

- children: 1.5 ml/kg
- adults: 1 ml/kg or 30–35 ml/kg body weight.

What are the biochemical markers that determine dehydration?

Dehydration is a fluid imbalance caused by inadequate intake or excessive losses. There are different biochemical markers that can identify and reveal the presence of dehydration. These markers are:

- urea/creatinine ration, which should be ≥ 0.15
- elevated levels of plasma sodium
- urine colour or specific urine gravity
- serum osmolarity.

Which categories of people are in danger of dehydration?

Hydration status, fluid balance and sufficient fluid depletion are important factors for the management of general health, and for the management of certain medical conditions and for the maintenance of physiological homoeostasis. Dehydration is linked with constipation, medication toxicity, renal failure, urinary tract infections, elevated body temperature, dizziness and general weakness. Those at risk of dehydration are:

- infants and young children, owing to poor intake or increased gastrointestinal losses
- older people or patients, owing to low fluid intake, blunted thirst response or poor food intake (anorexia, depression)
- people with eating and/or swallowing difficulties
- people with undiagnosed (or uncontrolled) diabetes mellitus and burns patients
- patients receiving diuretic drugs and laxatives or people with the symptoms of diarrhoea and/or vomiting
- patients suffering from pyrexia
- (mostly older) people with a physical immobility.

Further reading

Beaton GH, Milner J, McGuire V et al. (1983) Source of variance in 24-hour dietary recall data: Implications for nutrition study design and interpretation: Carbohydrate sources, vitamins, and minerals. American Journal of Clinical Nutrition 37(6): 986–95.

Chicago Dietetic Association/The South Shore Suburban Dietetic Association/Dieticians of Canada (2000) *Manual of Clinical Dietetics.* American Dietetic Association, Chicago, IL.

Dagenais GR, Yi Q, Mann JF *et al.* (2005) Prognostic impact of body weight and abdominal obesity in women and men with cardiovascular disease. *American Heart Journal* **149**(1): 54–60.

Hirsch J (1995) Role and benefits of carbohydrate in the diet: Key issues for future dietary guidelines. *American Journal of Clinical Nutrition* **61**(suppl. 4): S996–1000.

Kaplan RC, Heckbert SR and Furberg CD *et al.* (2002) Predictors of subsequent coronary events, stroke, and death among survivors of first hospitalized myocardial infarction. *Journal of Clinical Epidemiology* **55**: 654–64.

Kleiner SM (1999) Water: An essential but overlooked nutrient. *Journal of the American Dietetic Association* **99**: 200–206.

Lin XM, Zhang J, Zou ZY *et al.* (2008) Evaluation of serum transferrin receptor for iron deficiency in women of child-bearing age. *British Journal of Nutrition*: 1–5 (e-publication ahead of print).

Livingstone B, Black A (2003) Markers of the validity of reported intake. *Journal of Nutrition* **133**(suppl. 3): S895–920.

Mears E (1996) Outcomes of continuous process improvement of a nutritional care program incorporating serum prealbumin measurements. *Nutrition* **12**(7–8): 479–84.

Nyamdorj R, Qiao Q, Söderberg S *et al.* (2008) Comparison of body mass index with waist circumference, waist-to-hip ratio, and waist-to-stature ratio as a predictor of hypertension incidence in Mauritius. *Journal of Hypertension* **26**(5): 866–70.

Nyland J, Fried A, Maitra R *et al.* (2006) Wrist circumference is related to patellar tendon thickness in healthy men and women. *Clinical Imaging* **30**(5): 335–8.

Perry AC, Miller PC, Allison MD *et al.* (1998) Clinical predictability of the waist-to-hip ratio in assessment of cardiovascular disease risk factors in overweight, premenopausal women. *American Journal of Clinical Nutrition* **68**: 1022–7.

WHO Multicentre Growth Reference Study Group (2006) Reliability of anthropometric measurements in the WHO Multicentre Growth Reference Study. *Acta Paediatrica* **95**(3, suppl. 450): 38–46.

WHO Multicentre Growth Reference Study Group (2006) WHO child growth standards based on length/height, weight and age. *Acta Paediatrica* (suppl. 450): 76–85.

Woo J, Ho SC, Yu AL, Sham A (2002) Is waist circumference a useful measure in predicting health outcomes in the elderly? *International Journal of Obesity and Related Metabolic Disorders* **26**(10): 1349–55.

Zeman FJ, Ney DM (1996) *Applications in Medical Nutrition Therapy.* Prentice Hall, Upper Saddle River, NJ.

Chapter 2

Chapter 3

Malnutrition

Charilaos Dimosthenopoulos

What is malnutrition and how can it be classified?

'Malnutrition' is a general term for a medical condition caused by an improper or insufficient diet. The term usually refers to generally bad or faulty nutrition and is most often related to undernutrition. According to the World Health Organization (WHO), malnutrition is the 'cellular imbalance between supply of nutrients and energy and the body's demand for them to ensure growth, maintenance and specific functions', and is the greatest risk factor for illness and death worldwide. It can be associated with both undernutrition and overnutrition. Malnutrition and the state of deficiency or excess of energy, protein and other nutrients lead to measurable adverse effects on tissue, body function and appearance and clinical outcomes. There are different ways to classify malnutrition. Table 3.1 shows the classification of malnutrition as a loss of body weight based on a percentage of usual weight.

The Wellcome classification of severe malnutrition in children (a system for classifying protein–energy malnutrition in children based on percentage of expected weight-for-age and the presence or absence of oedema) is presented in Table 3.2.

What are the most common causes of malnutrition?

Anorexia, inadequate food intake or lack of food supplies and loss of appetite are probably the most common causes of malnutrition worldwide, especially in developing, but also in developed, countries. Anorexia can result from pathophysiological, psychological and general social problems. Different types of chronic and inflammatory diseases such as cystic fibrosis, chronic renal failure, stroke, Parkinson's disease, respiratory and orthopaedic problems, childhood malignancies, chronic inflammatory bowel diseases, fatigue, muscle weakness and difficulties with tasting, chewing and swallowing can

Table 3.1 Classification of malnutrition based on percentage of loss of body weight.

Type	Percentage
Mild	85–90%
Moderate	75–84%
Severe	<74%

lead to reduced food intake and malnutrition. Also, nausea and vomiting, which may result from certain diseases, and the use of certain drugs or specific treatments (chemotherapy, radiotherapy) may have a negative effect on appetite. Also, psychological factors such as anxiety and depression or the presence of dementia can cause malnutrition. Finally, malnutrition can have social causes, such as the institutionalisation of individuals (e.g. in hospitals, nursing homes), poverty and famine, poor food hygiene, inappropriate food supplies and the early cessation of breastfeeding.

What are the physical signs of both protein and energy malnutrition?

The most common physical signs of protein and energy malnutrition (PEM) are:

- weight loss and cachexia
- decreased subcutaneous tissue and reduction in muscle and body tissue mass, which can be most often observed in the legs, arms, buttocks and face
- oedemas
- neurological problems and abnormalities
- oral changes (red and usually swollen mouth, lips and gums)
- muscle cramp and pain
- skin changes (dry and peeling, frail, swollen, pale, loss of elasticity and poor healing)
- hair changes (dry and discoloured).

Table 3.2 The Wellcome classification of severe malnutrition in children.

| Weight for age (% of expected[a]) | Oedema | |
	Present	Absent
80–60	Kwashiorkor	Undernutrition
<60	Marasmic Kwashiorkor	Marasmus

[a] Expected weight-for-age by Harvard standards.

Is malnutrition synonymous with undernutrition?

'Malnutrition' is a general term that, although it encompasses overnutrition resulting from overeating or the excessive intake of nutrients (e.g. fat, simple sugars and carbohydrates), most often refers to undernutrition resulting from inadequate consumption, poor absorption or the excessive loss of nutrients and calories, regardless of whether any other specific nutrient is a limiting factor. On the other hand, malnutrition arises from deficiencies of specific nutrients or from diets based on inappropriate combinations or proportions of foods.

What is cachexia and what are its main symptoms?

Cachexia is a wasting syndrome, regulated by cytokines, and a condition of general ill health, malnutrition, undesired weight loss and physical weakness. Cachexia is associated with various chronic and end-stage diseases and medical conditions (e.g. metabolic acidosis, infectious diseases, autoimmune disorders and malignant conditions, such as various cancers, infections, AIDS, congestive heart failure, cystic fibrosis and Crohn's disease). It is characterised by changes in fat, protein and carbohydrate metabolism such as increased lipolysis, gluconeogenesis and protein turnover, glucose intolerance and hyperinsulinaemia, hyperlipidaemia, decreased plasma levels of branched-chain amino acids (BCAAs).

Cancer cachexia is one of the commonest types of cachexia, which describes a syndrome of progressive weight loss, anorexia and persistent erosion of host body cell mass, as a response to a malignant growth. It represents the clinical consequence of a chronic, systemic inflammatory response. The main symptoms of cancer cachexia, which is characterised by elevated levels of fibrinogen, are weakness, loss of appetite, muscle atrophy and fatigue.

Who is at risk of malnutrition?

Globally, malnutrition is the most important risk factor for illness and death and the main cause of more than half the deaths of children worldwide. Apart from infants and adolescents, who are very susceptible to malnutrition for various reasons, other categories of people at risk are:

- older people, in nursing homes or hospitals, and especially those who are suffering from long-term illnesses or chronic metabolic disorders
- poor people who are underfed or poorly fed
- people living in less-developed or developing countries of the world
- patients with neurological diseases such as dementia
- pregnant women
- people living in deprived socioeconomic circumstances, without adequate sanitation, education or means of preparing food
- individuals at risk of systemic infections.

Chapter 3

What are the symptoms and causes of Kwashiorkor?

Kwashiorkor and marasmus are the two different forms of protein and energy malnutrition. The main cause of this form of malnutrition is inadequate protein intake and the low concentration of essential amino acids. Kwashiorkor (from the West African word for 'displaced child') is a severe form of undernutrition, which develops in individuals on diets with a low protein/energy ratio. The main symptoms of Kwashiorkor are oedema, wasting, liver enlargement, hypoalbuminaemia, steatosis and the possible depigmentation of skin and hair.

What are the symptoms and causes of marasmus?

Marasmus (from the Greek word for 'to waste away') is the other form of malnutrition, which is caused by the inadequate intake of both protein and energy. It is a form of severe cachexia with weight loss as a result of wasting in infancy and childhood. The main symptoms of marasmus are severe wasting, with little or no oedema, minimal subcutaneous fat, severe muscle wasting and non-normal serum albumin levels.

What are the main clinical signs of the most common vitamin and mineral deficiencies?

The most common clinical signs of vitamin and mineral deficiencies are presented in Table 3.3.

Which screening tools should be used to detect malnutrition in the hospital setting?

Disease-related malnutrition is a common problem, which can be detected in nearly all health care settings. The prevalence of disease-related malnutrition is reported from various studies to range from 25–40% in hospital inpatients to 15–25% in home care units and 20–25% in nursing homes. Screening is essential, must be easy and fast and should be done as soon as patients are admitted, in order to define and validate whether they are at risk of malnutrition and what action should be taken.

The introduction of a malnutrition screening tool for hospital outpatients can play a crucial role in improving the detection of disease-related malnutrition. There are various nutrition screening tools, such as the Malnutrition Universal Screening Tool (MUST), Nutritional Risk Screening – 2002 (NRS-2002), Mini-Nutritional Assessment (MNA), Short Nutritional Assessment Questionnaire (SNAQ), Malnutrition Screening Tool (MST) and the Nutrition MedPass, which aim to determine nutritional status and predict the possible presence

Table 3.3 Most common clinical signs of vitamin and mineral deficiencies.

Vitamins/Minerals	Clinical signs
Calcium	Numbness, muscle aches (in extreme cases), rickets, fractures, muscle spasms
Magnesium	Irregular heart rhythms (arrhythmias), seizures, dizziness, weakness
Selenium	Impaired thyroid function, impaired cardiac function, enlarged heart
Zinc	Loss of taste
Vitamin D	Rickets, risk of fractures, low bone density and weak bones
Folic acid	Increased risk of specific birth defect (neural tube defect), elevated homocysteine levels, anaemia, fatigue
Vitamin C	Scurvy, poor appetite, digestion problems, bruising, slower healing of cuts
Beta-carotene (Vitamin A)	Eye damage (e.g. lack of night vision), dry skin
Vitamin B-6	Low red blood cell count (anaemia), low white blood cell count (neutropenia), poor appetite, trouble concentrating, reduced strength, hair loss, elevated homocysteine levels
Vitamin B-12	Pernicious anaemia, muscle weakness, confusion in older people, tingling in the hands/feet, elevated homocysteine levels
Vitamin E	Lack of coordination

of malnutrition, improve patient outcomes (e.g. weight status) and compliance and, finally, promote early nutritional therapy. According to the latest European Society of Parenteral and Enteral Nutrition (ESPEN) guidelines for nutritional screening, MUST is the most widely used screening tool for adults, mainly in the community, but also in hospitals settings, where NRS-2002 is the most appropriate tool for undernutrition detection, with an additional grading of severity of diseases. Both these tools have excellent reliability and a high level of validity. Apart from the above-mentioned tools, there is another one that concerns and is mainly used for older people. This tool is MNA, which includes physical and mental parameters and a dietary questionnaire, for the detection of undernutrition among older people, even in the early stages. The ESPEN guidelines state that there is, as yet, no universally accepted screening tool for children.

All these screening tools include the assessment of risk factors such as: difficulty in chewing and swallowing, presence of dysphagia, loss of appetite for more than three days, unintentional weight loss, levels of prealbumin and albumin, energy intake and the presence of pressure ulcers, multiple food allergies or intolerances, skin breakdown or intravenous nutrition (total parenteral nutrition or peripheral parenteral nutrition).

What are the main causes of hospital malnutrition?

The main causes of hospital malnutrition are usually related to the lack of:

- global interest in nutrition and/or poor recording of food intake in patient notes and inadequate referral to dietitians
- nutritional support
- practice guidelines and nationally agreed standards
- clearly defined responsibilities in planning and managing nutritional care
- sufficient educational level with regard to nutrition among all staff groups (medical and nursing)
- patients' influence and knowledge
- cooperation between different staff groups
- involvement by the hospital management.

What are the principal ways of treating a malnourished patient?

The treatment of a malnourished patient is determined by their general health, levels of weight loss and food intake and should follow the guidelines for the treatment of adult patients at risk of developing refeeding syndrome, a fatal medical condition that may affect malnourished and/or ill patients who receive an inappropriately high protein/calorie intake.

When normal food intake provides insufficient levels of energy and protein, additional nutrition can be given to the patient enterally or parenterally. When the gastrointestinal tract does not function properly, the fortification of food intake with protein, fat or carbohydrate oral supplements, mainly in powder or liquid form, the use of oral sip supplements, enteral nutrition through nasogastric tube or gastrostomy and, finally, central or peripheral parenteral nutrition can provide all of the macro- and micronutrients the patient needs to retain their lost weight and to meet their nutritional needs.

Further reading

Bavelaar JW, Otter CD, van Bodegraven AA *et al.* (2008) Diagnosis and treatment of (disease-related) in-hospital malnutrition: The performance of medical and nursing staff. *Clinical Nutrition* **27**(3): 431–8.

Edington J, Boorman J, Durrant E *et al.* (2000) Prevalence of malnutrition on admission to four hospitals in England: The Malnutrition Prevalence Group, *Clinical Nutrition* **19**(3): 191–5.

Ferguson M, Capra S, Bauer J, Banks M (1999) Development of a valid and reliable malnutrition screening tool for adult acute hospital patients. *Nutrition* **15**(6): 458–64.

Kondrup J, Allison SP, Elia M *et al.* (2002) Educational and Clinical Practice Committee, European Society of Parenteral and Enteral Nutrition (ESPEN). ESPEN guidelines for nutrition screening. *Clinical Nutrition* **22**(4): 415–21.

Livingstone C (2004) Refeeding syndrome and nutritional support. *Clinical Nutrition* **4**(5): 36–8.

Neelemaat F, Kruizenga HM, de Vet HCW *et al.* (2008) Screening malnutrition in hospital outpatients: Can the SNAQ malnutrition screening tool also be applied to this population? *Clinical Nutrition* **27**(3): 439–46.

Shetty P (2003) Malnutrition and undernutrition. *Medicine* **31**: 18–22.

Stratton RJ (2007) Pennington Lecture Malnutrition: Another health inequality? *Proceedings of the Nutrition Society* **66**: 522–9.

Stratton RJ, Hackston A, Longomore D *et al.* (2004) Malnutrition in hospital outpatients and inpatients: prevalence, concurrent validity and ease of use of the 'malnutrition universal screening tool' ('MUST') for adults. *British Journal of Nutrition* **92**(5): 799–808.

Volkert D, Berner YN, Berry E *et al.* (2006) ESPEN guidelines on enteral nutrition: Geriatrics. *Clinical Nutrition* **25**(2): 330–60.

World Health Organization (1999) *Management of Severe Malnutrition: A Manual of Physicians and Other Senior Health Workers.* WHO, Geneva.

Chapter 3

Chapter 4

Weight Management and Eating Disorders

Nikolaos Katsilambros and Charilaos Dimosthenopoulos

Prevention of obesity

With the term 'obesity', we characterise an abnormal or excessive accumulation of body fat, which constitutes a great threat to health. Obesity is a very serious health problem rather than a problem of appearance. Obesity, and more specifically the central type of obesity, which is characterised by excess fatty tissue around the abdominal region, is associated with an increased risk of developing diabetes and cardiovascular disease, and perhaps even 'the metabolic syndrome'.

What is the difference between an overweight and an obese patient?

Although, for the majority of people, the terms 'overweight' and 'obese' seem to be synonymous, there is a significant difference between them. Health professionals can determine whether a person is overweight or obese by combining their age and gender with the anthropometric parameters of their body weight, body mass index (BMI) and body fat mass. An adult who has a BMI of 25–29.9 kg/m^2 is said to be overweight, while an adult with a BMI in excess of 30 kg/m^2 is said to be obese. In the case of children and adolescents, the various BMI and weight ranges are different from those of adults, and the fact that normal levels of fat in the body vary depending on gender and age must be taken into account. In the case of children or teenagers, the various BMI and weight ranges are different from those for adults and take into consideration the normal differences in body fat, according to gender (boys or girls) and age group.

Table 4.1 Weight status categories and percentile ranges.

Weight status category	Percentile range
Underweight	Less than the 5th percentile
Healthy weight	5th percentile to less than the 85th percentile
At risk of overweight	85th to less than the 95th percentile
Overweight	Equal to or greater than the 95th percentile

Can body mass index be used in children?

BMI is a useful screening tool and the most widely used index for the identification of possible weight problems among children, although it is not usually considered a reliable indicator of body fatness in the individual as it fails to distinguish between lean body mass and fat. Certainly, from a public health and statistical perspective, BMI measurements of a population are still a very good indicator.

Thus, the relationship between BMI and body fatness varies according to body composition and proportions. The Centers for Disease Control and Prevention (CDC) and the American Academy of Pediatrics (AAP) recommend the use of BMI for the screening of overweight or obese children above the age of 2 years old. BMI for children and teens is combined with age growth charts (for either girls or boys). The growth charts show the weight status categories (underweight, healthy weight, at risk of overweight, overweight) for children and teens. BMI for age weight status categories and the corresponding percentiles are shown in Table 4.1.

Is there a genetic predisposition towards obesity?

The pathogenetic mechanism of obesity is still a big mystery, as there is still the question of the interaction between relevant environmental factors and genetic correlates in the development of the disease. In recent years, research into genetics has greatly increased our understanding of the mechanisms involved in the imbalance of the body weight and the body mass, and the features of genetic conditions such as Prader-Willi syndrome and Bardet-Biedl syndrome. Today we know that key genes, which are located on specific chromosomes (e.g. 2p, 3q, 5p, 6p, 7q, 10p, 11q, 17p and 20q), may influence many parameters related to energy intake and energy expenditure, and that they are associated with the basic metabolic rate, thermogenesis due to food intake and how active a person is generally inclined to be. Scientific findings on genetic predisposition to the development of obesity come from various studies on animals, and humans. A large number of studies between twins, adopted children and their families have shown that genetic factors play a significant role in the pathogenesis of obesity, while certain genes involved in pathways which regulate food intake and energy expenditure may play a role in predisposition to obesity. Obesity is most strongly related with:

- variations in the sequence of genes, e.g. in uncoupling proteins (UCPs), the adrenergic receptors, the peroxisome proliferator-activated receptor (PPRAs) and the leptin receptor (OBR)
- polymorphisms and mutations in various genes, which are responsible for the control of appetite by the hypothalamus; the metabolism; or the adipokine release predispose to obesity [e.g. the FTO gene, the TNF-α or the gene related to the synthesis of the melanocortin receptor or the proopiomelanocortin (POMC) gene that impairs the synthesis or structure of POMC-derived peptides].

In conclusion, it could be said that the development of obesity is partially determined by genes and genetic factors, but the environment (diet, activity, way of life, stress, etc.) influences its phenotypic expression.

What role does dietary fat intake play in the development of obesity?

The increase in fat intake of the modern diet and reduced physical activity are the two main causes of the development of obesity in industrialised countries. Fat is the most energy-dense nutrient in our diet, producing nine calories per gram, which is more than twice the calories derived from other macronutrients such as carbohydrates and proteins. At the same time, dietary fat is more efficiently metabolised and stored in body fat than carbohydrates are. Finally, although very fatty foods provide a high amount of calories, in parallel with an intense feeling of enjoyment and pleasure, they do not produce a strong feeling of satiety. For this reason they are usually over-consumed, which encourages the passive over-consumption of calories and the development of obesity by affecting the body's total energy balance. Over-consumption and the extra amount of dietary fat intake can lead to its storage in fat tissue (in percentage terms sometimes as high as 96%). Thus, an initial recommendation to lower dietary fat intake to initiate significant weight loss is reasonable and supported by scientific literature, experiments on animals and clinical studies in humans.

An increase in dietary fat intake leads to obesity in animals and has been associated with a higher prevalence of overweight and obesity in many human population studies. One of the main mechanisms through which dietary fat can contribute to the development of obesity is the regulation of leptin levels. Experiments have shown that an increased dietary fat intake results in central leptin resistance, whereas the restriction of dietary fat can lead to a partial improvement in leptin signalling, resulting in a spontaneous reduction in appetite and body weight. Of course, there is always the paradox of the modern diet, where the average fat content of the American diet is dropping (from 36% to 34%, according to the most recent National Health and Nutrition Examination Survey), but the weight of the average American continues to increase, mainly because the number of total calories continues to increase.

What is the role of sugar and carbohydrate intake in the development of obesity?

Carbohydrates represent the most essential energy fuel for the organism and play a very important role in our diet. They produce greater satiety, especially when they are in the form of complex high-fibre types, a better control of pre- and postprandial blood glucose levels and a higher dietary-induced thermogenesis, with a lower energy density (3.75 kcal/g (15.7 kJ/g), than fats (9 kcal/g, 37.68 kJ/g). The association between the intake of carbohydrates and obesity is still debateable. This relationship depends on the total amount consumed and energy requirements, as well as the type of carbohydrate and how refined or complex it is. For example, a high consumption of simple carbohydrates (in the form of non-starch polysaccharides) produces an imbalance on the blood glucose levels, a greater feeling of hunger and lower satiety and caloric over-consumption. These simple sugars, especially sucrose in refreshments and fructose in juices, have a direct effect on decreasing insulin resistance, increasing lipid levels and increasing body weight when consumed in large amounts.

On the other hand, a diet that is high in complex carbohydrates from fruits, vegetables, legumes and whole wheat and grain products provides a large amount of dietary fibre, which may play an important role in producing greater satiety and weight loss, while the parallel lowering of total-fat intake in the diet can also result in a spontaneous reduction in total energy (caloric) intake and weight loss in overweight and obese persons. During the last few decades, the low-carbohydrate and high-protein diets have become very popular, suggesting severe carbohydrate restriction as the absolute solution to the obesity problem. It is known that this restriction of carbohydrate intake initially mobilises glycogen stores in the liver and induces the production of ketone bodies (ketogenesis) through the use of free fatty acids instead of glucose, as energy fuel, and increased diuresis.

Is the overconsumption of calories responsible for the development of obesity?

There are different causes for the development of obesity, which are related to genetics, human biology, hormones and environmental factors. An imbalance between energy intake and energy expenditure is consider the most important. When we consume more calories than we expend for our daily needs (basal metabolic rate, thermogenic processes and activity), this extra energy is stored in the body, mainly as fat stored in fat tissue, in order to be used later as an energy fuel. Therefore, apart from the quality of the diet and the proportion of fat, protein and carbohydrates, the total quantity of energy intake and energy consumed is most important for the energy balance of the body.

Treatment of obesity

What are the characteristics of an ideal weight-loss diet?

An ideal dietary weight-reducing programme must contain all the food groups, without excluding any of them (e.g. low-carbohydrate diets). It is a programme that includes daily servings of fruits and vegetables (raw or cooked), fat-free or low-fat milk and milk products and servings from starchy foods (e.g. bread, rice, pasta, cereals) and potatoes, legumes, adequate protein sources such as lean meat, poultry, fish, beans, eggs and nuts, with a certain amount of fat, mainly in the form of monounsaturated olive oil. It is obvious that an ideal weight-reducing diet could be described and based on the Eatwell Plate from the Food Standards Agency.

In any diet, adequate protein, derived from both plant sources and lean sources of animal protein, is essential to help spare lean body mass. In weight-reducing diet programmes, protein intake should be 0.8–1.5 g/kg (0.36–0.68 g/lb) of body weight per day. Alcohol consumption, although generally recommended to the healthy population, not only increases the number of calories in a diet but also is associated with the development of obesity, in epidemiological studies and in experimental studies. For this reason, alcohol in a hypocaloric diet would provide unneeded calories, displacing more nutritious foods.

At the same time, an ideal dietary programme should be characterised by variety, proportionality, flexibility and personalisation and should cover the nutritional and energy needs of the dieter, according to their age, gender, resting metabolic rate, health status, level of physical activity and their lifestyle. The total reduction in calories should not exceed 500–1000 kcal/day (2093–4189 kJ/day), in order to achieve a weight loss of 0.5–1 kg/week (1.1–2.2 lb/week). Finally, during weight loss, attention should be given to maintaining an adequate intake of vitamins and minerals (e.g. iron and calcium).

What are the very low calorie diets? Are they useful and healthy choices? Who should follow them?

During the 1970s and early 1980s, very low calorie diets (VLCDs) became very popular, mainly because of their immediate weight-reducing results. VLCDs are very strict dietary programmes that provide a very low-energy intake of 400–800 kcal (1675–3349 kJ) and a total protein intake of 45–100 g per day, in the form of regular foods and meals, but also as specially prepared liquid formulas. Being so low in energy, VLCDs are severely restricted in terms of their carbohydrate and fat intake A multivitamin supplement was included in regular foods, rather than a special formula, in order to provide adequate amounts of vitamins and minerals. People on a VLCD must drink over two litres of water and they can drink other non-caloric fluids (tea, coffee or others).

These diets are advised for a short period (no more than three months) and only under medical supervision. They can be dangerous, as they are not nutritionally balanced diets and they may produce certain nutritional and electrolyte deficiencies, lean body mass loss or development of medical problems (e.g. gallstones). For this reason, these programmes are not suitable for all overweight or obese people, but only to obese patients that cannot lose weight through conventional methods and diets of modest caloric restriction, and to patients with certain medical problems, in whom a rapid weight loss is indicated. They are often prescribed to the morbidly obese patient, under medical supervision, prior to their undergoing bariatric surgery, and during and post-surgery, in order to reduce complications.

Are high-protein diets more appropriate for the treatment of obesity?

High-protein diets are the most popular type of exclusion diets used in the weight-control industry. The higher intake of protein and the severe restriction of carbohydrates in the diet, through the exclusion of fruits, starchy foods and legumes, had been considered the best solution for obesity. It is true that protein provides specific benefits in the diet that are useful during a weight-reducing diet programme. First of all, protein produces more diet-induced thermogenesis, than fat and carbohydrate, increasing energy expenditure. Moreover, meals containing protein (meat products, poultry, cheese, egg whites, etc.) induce satiety, prolong the feeling of fullness and depress hunger. Protein metabolism produces higher diuresis, which contributes to a larger initial weight loss. A low-carbohydrate programme contributes to a lower intake of overall calories, to a lower plasma insulin level and improved insulin sensitivity, which leads to a higher fat oxidation and utilisation of fat as energy fuel, by promoting ketosis, which also leads to weight loss.

These dietary programmes seem to be effective and to contribute to weight loss only in the short term, while in the long term they have almost the same effect as low-fat and high-carbohydrate diets. Also, they can be dangerous, in the case of long-term application, as they allow and promote the consumption of high-fat and high-salt protein foods, which can lead to higher levels of cholesterol and increased levels of blood pressure, and prohibit the consumption of vitamin and mineral-rich food sources, such as fruits and starchy vegetables and cereals.

Is water beneficial for the treatment of obesity?

Water is a vital component of any healthy diet (including weight-reducing programmes), as it is essential for the preservation of life and the regulation of the body's temperature and metabolism. Adequate water intake has direct and indirect effects on the regulation of body weight. Drinking a lot of water, which is always advised during weight-reducing diets before a main meal can help to fill the stomach, decrease appetite and determine the total amount of food intake, resulting in an increase of the chance of weight loss. It also helps to prevent dehydration, the excretion of ketones and other products and the regulation of intestinal function. The intake of water can influence the amount of fat burned by the body, increase the metabolic rate [it is estimated that drinking 500 ml (17.5 fl oz) of water results in an increase of the metabolic rate of around 30%] and the daily energy expenditure, through water-induced thermogenesis. Indirectly, water intake can play a role in the treatment of obesity, especially in the case of childhood obesity. In addition, adequate water intake is indicated because fasting results in an increase of serum uric acid. Children can benefit from drinking water, which is calorie-free and decreases thirst without adding calories, and so avoids their taking extra calories from drinking sugary soft drinks and fruits juices, which increase total energy intake during meals.

When is a nutritional supplement beneficial during a weight-reducing programme?

The use of a multivitamin or a mineral supplement is not always needed during a weight-reducing programme. A diet programme with a modest reduction of energy intake, which includes all the food groups, can still provide the dieter, in most cases, with all of the necessary vitamins and minerals. In the cases of stricter programmes, when the caloric level is lower than 1200 kcal (5024 kJ), or in the presence of specific groups of people (e.g. adolescents, lactating women), a supplement is usually necessary since the food intake may be insufficient. The most commonly used supplements are those of iron, sodium, potassium, magnesium, phosphorus and calcium. Apart from the known supplements, a wide variety of other nutritional supplements are usually proposed during the diet. Fish oils (good sources of omega 3, which improve glucose-insulin metabolism and cholesterol levels), conjugated linoleic acid (CLA), chitosan, L-carnitine, but also herbs, such as the dangerous ephedra (also known as ma huang, which has been withdrawn recently because it has been linked with fatal complications such as liver failure), psyllium (a soluble fibre), green tea (*Camellia sinensis*), capsaicin (*Capsicum frutescens*) and others are some of the 'natural' supplements that are suggested as promoting weight reduction. All of these should only be administrated with medical approval and should be a part of a balanced weight-reducing dietary programme.

What is the role of exercise in the treatment of obesity?

Exercise is considered a cornerstone of weight loss and weight maintenance. It represents the second component of energy balance, which is the output or the energy expenditure that is necessary to achieve a positive energy balance and weight loss. Body weight is determined by the balance between energy intake and energy expenditure, and weight loss can only be achieved by decreasing energy intake and/or increasing physical activity.

The benefits of exercise are numerous and are associated with the physiological, the psychological and the biochemical aspects of weight loss. Physical activity plays a crucial role in the minimisation of the decrease in the basal metabolic rate (BMR) because of the energy restriction that occurs during a weight-reducing diet. It is also essential for the prevention of the loss of lean body mass, as well as for reducing fat mass, promoting a healthy heart, having a better control of blood glucose levels and a higher insulin sensitivity and improving the lipid profile levels (enhancement of high-density lipoprotein, or HDL). Exercise contributes to the suppression of the appetite, improves the psychological status of the dieter and is extremely important for the maintenance of any weight loss.

The American Heart Association recommends at least 30–45 minutes of moderate/intense physical activity (e.g. walking) as many days as possible in the week, while other foundations, such as the Institute of Medicine, recommend an even greater frequency of moderate/intense exercise, which should last approximately 60 minutes per day (which can be as intermittent activity throughout the day, rather than a single period of exercise). The type of exercise, its the frequency and intensity are strongly related to the severity and morbidity of obesity, the mobility of the obese patient and their motivation and so its type and level of intensity should be specific to the individual patient's needs and physical ability.

Diet and weight control

What are the lower levels of calorie intake for men and women?

It is widely accepted that in order to achieve the best weight reduction, a reduction in calorie intake of 500–1000 kcal (2093–4187 kJ) per day will help to achieve a healthy and gradual, weekly weight loss. Although many popular diets suggest a very drastic decrease in energy intake, according to the literature, the energy allowance should be lower than 1000–1200 kcal/day (4187–5024 J/day) for women and 1200–1600 kcal/day (5024–6699 J/day) for men.

Are there nutritional supplements appropriate for weight loss?

Numerous nutritional supplements claim to promote weight reduction in parallel with a low-calorie dietary plan. According to their function, these supplements have been organised by the Food & Drug Administration into the following categories:

- increased energy consumption: supplements such as ephedra, bitter orange, guarana, caffeine, country mallow, yarbe mate

- increased satiety: guar gum, psyllium, glucomannan
- increased lipid oxidation: L-carnitine, hydroxycitric acid, green tea, vitamin B$_5$, liquorice, pyruvate, CLA (conjugated linoleic acid – naturally occurring fatty acid, which is found in meat, cheese and dairy products)
- decreased lipid absorption: chitosan
- various ways of function: laminaria, spirulina, apple cider vinegar, etc.

Although for all the above supplements there are various studies and scientific findings on their role in lipid oxidation, total energy consumption and the feeling of fullness, it is generally accepted that none of them can play a dramatic role in total weight reduction and for this reason they are not considered essential in weight-reducing programmes.

Dietary management of patients after bariatric surgery

When is bariatric surgery recommended for treating obesity?

It is accepted that the weight of the majority of overweight or obese patients is a low to moderate health risk. Therefore, bariatric surgery treatment, which is very popular nowadays, is not the proper solution for all cases of obesity. The indications of bariatric surgery can be summarised as follows:

$$BMI \geq 40\,kg/m^2$$

or with the presence of obesity-related disorders, such as diabetes, high blood pressure, sleep apnoea and/or other problems:

$$BMI \geq 35\,kg/m^2$$

and a history of unsuccessful weight loss by non-surgical means, such as diet, exercise and lifestyle modifications, i.e. anyone with a BMI of between 35 and 40 kg/m^2.

What is the main dietary advice for a patient after ring insertion?

Ring insertion (also known as gastric band insertion) is one of the most popular types of treatment for morbid obesity. The first phase of the postoperative diet is the clear liquids phase (apple juice, orange juice, water, flat diet soft drinks, sugar-free jelly, low-fat soup, etc.). When these liquids are well tolerated, the patients pass to the second phase, which includes semi-liquid foods and drinks and lasts for one to two weeks. The patient receives all the foods in a similar consistency to that of thinned mashed potatoes. During this phase, the patient is fed with skimmed or semi-skimmed milk, blended soups (made with skimmed milk instead of water, to increase the protein content), blended fruit, shakes made with skimmed milk and light/non-fat yogurt and blended meat, creamy soups, mashed potatoes made with skimmed milk and sugar-free yogurt. This phase lasts for approximately two weeks, according to the degree of tolerance. Immediately afterwards comes the third phase, of the semi-solid diet.

This diet consists of low-fat cottage cheese, cooked, peeled vegetables, boiled or canned fruits in natural juice, boiled eggs, chopped lean meat, skimmed or semi-skimmed milk, unsweetened instant breakfast (e.g. porridge oats), sugar-free, low-fat yogurt and boiled chicken. The last phase is the low-fat solids diet. This is low in fat and sugar, avoids carbonated and caffeinated drinks but includes plenty of other, non-alcoholic, fluids [as much as 1500–1800 ml (52.5–63 fl oz) according to the patient's tolerance]. The patient must add one new food at a time, must chew all food very well and sip only limited amounts of liquids with their meal, and if necessary must take a vitamin/mineral supplement to cover any nutritional needs.

What is the main dietary advice for a patient after a Roux-en-Y operation?

The Roux-en-Y gastric bypass is a process which involves the creation of a small stomach pouch and the bypass of the distal stomach and the proximal small bowel, and is a very drastic way for weight reduction for morbidly obese patients. This operation can often lead to long-term iron, calcium, vitamin B_{12} and vitamin D deficiencies. The postoperative diet is liquid-based for the first week. On day one post-surgery the patient must drink in small sips and wait in-between sips for some minutes and avoid taking more that 100 ml (3.5 fl oz) at once, while the total fluid intake should be at least 2000 ml (70 fl oz) per day. For days 2–6 they must be on a liquid diet, with sugar-free fruit juice, skimmed milk, clear soups and vegetable juices, and if necessary on protein drinks and supplements. For the second week (days 7–13), they should be on a puréed diet, which has a thicker consistency. This diet includes yoghurt, porridge, skimmed or semi-skimmed milk, soups, scrambled egg, pureed meat and blended vegetables, fruits and vegetable juices.

Adequate hydration is important. Patients are advised to drink slowly and not during meals. In weeks 2–3, they must return gradually to the soft diet (i.e. in which all the foods included are of a soft texture), always according to their tolerance. This diet includes bread, lean meat, fat spreads, low-fat cheese, eggs, yoghurt, soups, fish, chicken, mashed potatoes, boiled vegetables or even a sorbet. At this stage, the patient must drink enough fluids, avoid fat when cooking, chew meats well and add any new food slowly, to avoid bloating or nausea. Finally, four weeks after the operation, the patient is ready to progress to a regular diet, with 5–6 small meals per day, as long as the previous diets have been tolerated. Adequate protein intake is still essential and for this reason protein supplements may be necessary. Finally, adequate fluid is essential to maintain hydration and the patient needs approximately 6–8 cups of fluid per day.

How much protein and fluid should be given to the patient after the operation?

The most frequent nutritional problems that appear after bariatric surgery are dehydration, protein malnutrition and vitamin/mineral deficiency.

Fluids

Dehydration is often present after almost all types of surgery, mostly owing to limited fluid intake. Especially in cases of gastric bypass, patients have difficulty in getting the appropriate amount of fluid because of the limited content of the stomach. The symptoms of sweating, diarrhoea and vomiting, in parallel with greater faecal production, enhance fluid loss. There are no specific recommendations for fluid intake, but patients are advised to drink plenty of fluid, using the sense of thirst and the quantity and colour of urine as markers of sufficient hydration. Nutritional fluids (e.g. juices, low-fat milk) are preferable, since they provide energy and protein apart from hydration, while non-nutritional fluids are best avoided or at least restricted to between meals.

Protein

According to recent research, the most important macronutrient to take after bariatric surgery (e.g. gastric bypass surgery) is protein. Protein, in contrast to fat or carbohydrate, does not change gastric transit time significantly, while at the same time it is essential for tissue repair and growth after a major surgical procedure. In these cases, a high-protein diet contributes to the faster healing of the trauma, the maintenance of an increased basal metabolic rate and the stimulation of the protein synthesis. A protein intake of 60–90 g/day is recommended for the postoperative period through the consumption of high-protein foods or the use of sugar-free fluid protein supplements, which provide all the adequate essential amino acids, but also vitamins and minerals, which were malabsorbed in the postoperative period. Protein is important even after recovery, as it continues to provide adequate thermogenic action, in order to lose weight or to sustain previous weight loss.

Fad diets

What are fad diets?

When we say 'fad diets' we are usually referring to a wide variety of popular diets that mainly promote energy- or nutrient-restricted eating plans that exclude certain nutrients (e.g. low-carbohydrate diets). Therefore, fad diets are usually both unhealthy and insufficient, especially for children, and for the majority of adults. Diets such as the Cabbage Soup Diet, the South Beach Diet, the Hollywood Diet or the Grapefruit Diet are well promoted and commercialised, through books, magazines and TV series. Almost all of them are not based on scientific evidence and studies but on pseudo-scientific claims and are considered non-clinical dietary programmes that can even be harmful. They promote rapid weight loss by increasing diuresis and use of fat stores as energy fuel, through ketosis, and finally they overemphasise one food or type of food, banning a specific food or food group or suggesting that a specific food or product can increase the body's chemistry. They usually lack sufficient energy, protein and certain fat-soluble vitamins and minerals, which are essential for the maintenance of the total health status of the obese or overweight patient.

Anorexia nervosa and bulimia nervosa

How can we help the anorexic patient nutritionally?

Nutritional intervention, by a scientific group of specialists, is essential for the total health management of an anorexic patient. The restoration of normal nutrition, the prevention of muscle and bone loss, the increased energy intake level, the gradual weight gain and the normalised hormonal function are the main nutritional interventions needed, in the case of anorexia nervosa, in parallel with psychotherapeutic treatment. For all the above, it is necessary to provide nutritional support to these people, who are considered patients. First of all, a weight-gain goal of 0.5–1.0 kg/week (1.1–2.2 lb/week) is regarded as the optimum and is usually set by the doctor or the clinical dietitian. In cases of patients who weigh less than 45 kg (99 lb) and are severely malnourished, an initial calorie intake of 1400–1500 kcal/day (5862–6280 kJ/day) is considered a starting level of refeeding, in order to reduce the chances of stomach pain, bloating, fluid retention or heart failure and to reduce the patient's anxiety of becoming 'overweight', which is the main cause of the disorder.

In certain cases, when either extreme weight loss, a critical medical condition of the anorexic patient or refusal of feeding is present, tube or enteral feeding, preferably through a nasogastric tube, may be required. In these cases, in order to avoid fluid or electrolyte disturbances, tube feeding should have a slow flow (i.e. the rate of fluid going through the tube should be a low one), while the total fluid chart, electrolyte levels and blood glucose concentration must be carefully monitored. In the case of life-threatening situations, a patient can be fed intravenously for a short period, until oral or nasogastric feeding become possible.

What type of nutrients should be given to someone with anorexia nervosa?

Anorexics, owing to their decreased food intake and extreme weight loss, are at increased risk of vitamin and mineral deficiency. Nutrient deficiencies (e.g. vitamin abnormalities) may contribute to muscle mass catabolism, tissue damage (hair loss, bone density) and various cognitive difficulties (such as poor judgement, memory loss, other psychiatric conditions) and should be corrected through dietary intervention and supplementation. Planning the diet of a person with anorexia nervosa should consider the following macro- and micronutrients and ensure an adequate intake of:

- protein, to prevent and treat muscle mass loss
- carbohydrates, to avoid erratic weight changes
- fat and essential fatty acids
- nutrients necessary to support bone mineral density (calcium, vitamin D, magnesium)
- other minerals such as iron and zinc (zinc deficiency may cause altered taste as well as a variety of neuropsychiatric symptoms)
- fat-soluble vitamins (A, E, D, K).

A very important phase in the treatment of an anorexic is the refeeding period, especially for patients with a very low BMI, when a number of serious complications may occur, and dietary and medical monitoring is highly recommended. During this phase, a wide range of electrolyte disturbances (e.g. hypokalaemia, hypocalcaemia and hypomagnesaemia), referred to as 'refeeding syndrome', and renal or hepatic impairment, may occur. The consequences of this procedure can be minimised by avoiding an initial excessive protein intake, by giving the patient relatively small amounts of food and by increasing the quantities of all the nutrients progressively.

What are the main nutritional dangers in bulimia nervosa?

Bulimia nervosa is a serious, even life-threatening, and difficult-to-overcome eating disorder, in which patients are preoccupied with their weight, body fat and body shape. Bulimics usually judge themselves severely and produce episodes of bingeing and purging. Physical complications and dangers of bulimia nervosa often include imbalance in electrolytes (sodium, chloride and potassium abnormalities), gastrointestinal problems and oesophagus inflammation, constipation, bloating or nausea, anaemia, heart problems, tooth decay and gum problems, absence of a period and finally, in the most severe cases, death.

What is the role of a dietitian in the treatment of anorexia and bulimia nervosa?

The dietitian is one of the professionals who can contribute, as part of a scientific team, to the treatment of people with eating disorders. Eating disorders, such as anorexia and bulimia nervosa, have physiological, but mostly psychological, causes and require professional management and knowledge of the nutritional and health aspects of the illness. Anorexia nervosa involves extreme dietary behaviour, weight loss, electrolyte imbalance and increased nutritional requirements. The role of a clinical dietitian in the treatment of anorexia nervosa is crucial, for it is they who:

- collect the nutritional and behavioural information
- assess the level of undernutrition and of nutrient deficiencies, providing these data to the other members of the team
- try to establish a normal food intake
- incorporate a wider variety of food items in the daily dietary intake of the patient
- discuss and educate the anorexic on the adoption of a healthy and well-balanced meal plan.

Further reading

Anderson JW, Konz EC, Jenkins DJA (2000) Health advantages and disadvantages of weight-reducing diets: A computer analysis and critical review. *Journal of the American College of Nutrition* **19**(5): 578–90.

Astrup A, Meinert Larsen T, Harper A (2004) Atkins and other low-carbohydrate diets: Hoax or an effective tool for weight loss? *Lancet* **364**(9437): 897–9.

Astrup A, Toubro S, Raben A, Skov AR (1997) The role of low fat diets and fat substitutes in body weight management. What have we learned from clinical studies? *Journal of the American Dietetic Association* **97**(suppl. 7): S82–7.

Bennett W (1987) Dietary treatment of obesity. *Annals of the New York Academy of Sciences* **499**: 250–63.

Berkowitz VJ (2000) A view on high-protein, low-carb diets. *Journal of the American Dietetic Association* **100**(11): 1300, 1302–3.

Boschmann M, Steiniger J, Hille U *et al.* (2003) Water-induced thermogenesis. *Journal of Clinical Endocrinology and Metabolism* **88**: 6015–19.

Chakravarthy MV, Booth FW (2004). Eating, exercise, and 'thrifty' genotypes: Connecting the dots toward an evolutionary understanding of modern chronic diseases. *Journal of Applied Physiology* **96**(1): 3–10.

Dansinger ML, Gleason JA, Griffith JL *et al.* (2005) Comparison of the Atkins, Ornish, Weight Watchers, and Zone diets for weight loss and heart disease risk reduction: A randomized trial. *Journal of the American Medical Association* **293**(1): 43–53.

Dugan SA (2008) Exercise for preventing childhood obesity. *Physical Medicine and Rehabilitation Clinics of North America* **19**(2): 205–16.

Foster GD, Wyatt HR, Hill JO *et al.* (2000) A randomized trial of a low-carbohydrate diet for obesity. *New England Journal of Medicine* **348**(21): 2082–90.

Loos RJF, Bouchard C (2003) Obesity: Is it a genetic disorder? *Journal of International Medicine* **254**: 401–25.

Mayor S (2000) Researcher criticised for comments on the Atkins diet. *British Medical Journal* **327**(7412): 414.

Mei Z, Grummer-Strawn LM, Pietrobelli A *et al.* (2002) Validity of body mass index compared with other body-composition screening indexes for the assessment of body fatness in children and adolescents. *American Journal of Clinical Nutrition* **75**(6): 978–85.

Chapter 4

National Institutes of Health (1998) Clinical guidelines on the identification, evaluation, and treatment of overweight and obesity in adults: The evidence report. *Obesity Research* **6**(suppl. 2): S51–209.

Rolls BJ, Bell EA (2000) Dietary approaches to the treatment of obesity. *The Medical Clinics of North America* **84**(2): 401–18, vi.

Samaha FF, Iqbal N, Seshadri P *et al.* (2003) A low-carbohydrate as compared with a low-fat diet in severe obesity. *New England Journal of Medicine.* **348**(21): 2074–81.

Skender ML, Goodrick GK, Reeves RS *et al.* (1996) Comparison of two-year weight loss trends in behavioural treatments of obesity: Diet, exercise and combination interventions. *Journal of the American Dietetic Association* **96**(4): 342–6.

Sumithran P, Proietto J (2008) Safe year-long use of a very-low-calorie diet for the treatment of severe obesity. *Medical Journal of Australia* **188**(6): 366–8.

Tourbo S, Astrup A (1997) Randomised comparisons of diets of maintaining obese subjects' weight after major weight loss: Ad lib, low fat, high carbohydrated diet v fixed energy intake. *British Medical Journal* **314**(7073): 29–34.

Truby H, Baic S, deLooy A *et al.* (2006) Randomised controlled trial of four commercial weight loss programmes in the UK: Initial findings from the BBC 'diet trials'. *British Medical Journal* **332**(7553): 1309–14.

Chapter 4

Chapter 5

Diabetes

Nikolaos Katsilambros and Charilaos Dimosthenopoulos

Diabetes mellitus

Is the diabetic diet a strict or a healthy diet?

Before the discovery of insulin, in 1921, the recommendations for the appropriate diet for diabetes used to suggest a strict, monotonous and rigid diet, with very high percentages of fat and protein and very low percentages of carbohydrates. This made it very difficult for diabetic subjects to adhere to these recommendations. Over the years, these recommendations have been adjusted, mainly because of the availability of insulin and new medications, as well as because prolongation of the life of the diabetic person is accompanied by an increase in cardiovascular disease. Nowadays, the diet for diabetes is synonymous with a healthy diet for the general population, with a wider variety of nutritional options and more complex (or slowly absorbed) carbohydrate-rich foods in the daily dietary plan.

What are the primary dietary goals for type 1 diabetics?
What are the different suggestions for children and adults?

Type 1 diabetes, formerly called 'juvenile diabetes' or 'insulin-dependent diabetes', is usually diagnosed in children and adolescents. In type 1 diabetes, the beta cells of the pancreas no longer secrete insulin. It is treated only with insulin. The primary dietary goals for people with type 1 diabetes are the:

- maintenance of optimal metabolic outcomes and blood glucose levels
- reduction of the risk of complications of diabetes (e.g. macrovascular disease, vascular disease) and to treat them
- improvement of general health, through healthy food choices and physical activity

- modification of the person's nutrient intake and lifestyle, as appropriate, for the prevention and treatment of obesity, dyslipidaemia, cardiovascular disease, hypertension and nephropathy
- coverage of the individual's nutritional needs, according to personal and cultural preferences and lifestyle and their energy and nutritional needs
- maintenance of normal body weight.

What are the primary dietary goals for people with type 2 diabetes?

Type 2 diabetes, formerly called 'adult-onset diabetes' or 'non-insulin-dependent diabetes', is the most common type of diabetes. The onset of type 2 diabetes can be at any age – even during childhood – and is mainly caused by obesity. Type 2 diabetes usually begins with insulin resistance, a condition in which fat, muscle and liver cells do not use insulin properly. The dietary goals for people with type 2 diabetes are almost the same with those given for type 1. The main difference is related to the aetiology of this type of diabetes, which is generally combined with the presence of overweight or obesity. For this reason, one of the basic pieces of dietary advice for type 2 is weight loss, when appropriate, and the maintenance of a healthy weight through the combination of a caloric deficit, according to the specific energy and dietary needs of the individual, and an increased level of daily physical activity. Increased physical activity by people with type 2 diabetes improves glycaemia, decreases insulin resistance and reduces cardiovascular risk, independently of body weight changes. Individuals with type 2 diabetes are advised to have at least 150 min/week of moderate/intense aerobic physical activity, distributed over at least three days and with no more than two consecutive days without physical activity. Resistance training is also effective in improving glycaemia. People with type 2 diabetes are encouraged to perform resistance exercises three times a week.

Is it useful to use a glycaemic index? Should the diabetic diet include glycaemic-rich foods?

The glycaemic index (GI) is a useful tool for the management of blood glucose in people with diabetes and as a means of calculating the physiological effect of carbohydrates on blood glucose levels. It provides information which can assist people with diabetes in many ways but mainly in the adoption of healthy eating and the planning of healthy meals. The GI ranks carbohydrate-rich foods by how much they raise blood glucose levels compared to a standard food (which is usually glucose or white bread) and helps in the implementation of the guidelines for the nutritional management of diabetes mellitus.

A GI which is 70 or more is considered high; a GI of 56–69, medium; of 55 or less, low. A low-GI food causes a small rise, while a high-GI food results in a higher rise. The GI for foods such as whole wheat bread, legumes (lentils, chickpeas, baked beans), oatmeal and pasta is low (below 55), and high (70 or more) for foods such as white bread, bagels, corn flakes, short-grain rice, certain types of potato and French fries/chips. For people with diabetes, it is preferable to consume mainly foods with a low GI; however, it is difficult to avoid the ones with higher GI, as they are present in many dishes and meals.

What is the difference between the glycaemic index and the glycaemic load?

The GI, as mentioned above, is a numerical system of calculating the level of the rise of blood glucose after the consumption of a carbohydrate-rich food: the higher the GI number, the greater the postprandial blood sugar rise. The glycaemic load (GL) is a ranking system for carbohydrate content in food portions based on their GI and their portion size. This means that the GL is an alternative way to measure the effect of the consumption of carbohydrates that, while taking the GI into account, provides a better picture than the GI gives alone. Generally, the GI value shows how rapidly a particular carbohydrate, from a specific food item, turns into blood sugar, without providing any information of how much of that carbohydrate is in a serving of a particular food item. This information can be given by the GL. It is generally accepted that both figures, taken in tandem, are useful as in isolation neither gives the full picture. Foods with a low GL almost always have a low GI, while foods with an intermediate or high GL can have a very low or very high GI. Also, a high-GI food consumed in small quantities would give almost the same effect on blood glucose as larger quantities of a low-GI food.

Can people with diabetes consume sugar-free products? Are all the so-called light products appropriate for them?

There is a wide range of sugar substitutes that are used by the food industry instead of sucrose in sugar-free products. Polyols is one category of these substitutes which are widely used as sugar-free sweeteners. They belong to carbohydrates, although they are not sugars. The most common are sorbitol, xylitol, maltitol, isomalt, lactitol, mannitol and erythritol. These substances provide 0.2–3 kcal/g (0.84–12.56 kJ/g), while sugar (sucrose) provides approximately 4 kcal/g (16.75 kJ/g). Food products with polyols contain fewer calories and produce a lower, or even no, blood glucose rise, as they are partially absorbed. There are various studies on subjects with diabetes which have shown that sugar alcohols produce a lower postprandial glucose response than sucrose or glucose do and that polyols offer diabetics a low energy intake. At the same time, there are many other artificial sweeteners, such as acesulfame potassium, aspartame, saccharin and sucralose, that are used in very small amounts, as they are more than 200 times sweeter than sucrose, and for this reason they are considered calorie-free sweeteners. People with diabetes can consume sugar-free products, as they contain fewer calories than regular foods, but they must be aware of the type of sweetener used in any specific food product and also avoid overconsumption. Some can lead to health problems (e.g. Food & Drug Administration warns of the potential laxative effects of the excessive consumption of sorbitol or mannitol), and to the overconsumption of calories and carbohydrates.

As far as it concerns the wide range of 'light' products that can be found on the market, it should be noted that they are not totally accepted and appropriate for people with diabetes, as many still contain a high percentage of calories derived from fat or other sugar substitutes, such as fructose, which have the same caloric load as sucrose. This means that their consumption can still increase body weight, or even blood glucose levels.

What types of fibre are appropriate for diabetic subjects and from which food sources can we take them?

Dietary fibre is a very important part of the diet for people with diabetes. Fibre from foods can be soluble or insoluble. Of these two types, it is recommended that people with diabetes should consume mainly soluble fibre. A daily intake of soluble fibre (5–10 g/d) is recommended from oats, barley, legumes or purified fibre sources – such as psyllium, pectin and guar – and can reduce serum cholesterol by 5–10%. Purified soluble fibre sources reduce blood glucose responses and have been associated with improved blood glucose control. However, soluble fibre content alone is not a reliable indicator of a food's metabolic effect. Research indicates that the insoluble fibre content of whole foods is more closely related to their GI than the soluble fibre content is. This is consistent with data from epidemiological studies, which suggest that insoluble fibres from cereals may reduce the risk of coronary heart disease and type 2 diabetes by up to 30% for each 10 g increment in intake.

- Total dietary fibre intake of at least 25–35 g/d from a variety of sources is advised for adults. For children, 5 g plus 1 g per year of age is suggested as a general guide.
- Including more foods and food combinations that combine cereal fibre with low GI may be helpful to optimise health outcomes for people with diabetes.

Do people with diabetes require less protein than others do?

Current evidence indicates that individuals with diabetes have similar protein requirements as the general population – about 0.8–1 g/kg per day (0.36–0.45 g/lb) and that their usual protein intake (15–20% of energy) should not be modified. In the case of overweight or obese people with diabetes, high-protein diets may produce short-term weight loss and improve glycaemia, but they are not recommended as an appropriate method of weight loss. The long-term effect on, and any complications for, the management of diabetes of a protein intake of over 20% of total calorie intake has not been established. Protein plays a role in stimulating insulin secretion, but excessive intake should be avoided, as it may contribute to the pathogenesis of diabetic nephropathy. Some evidence suggests eating vegetable protein, rather than animal protein, is better for reducing serum cholesterol and managing nephropathy.

Recommendations

- Protein intake should be at least 0.8–1 g/kg (0.36–0.45 g/lb) per day.
- In diabetic nephropathy the protein allowance is less than 0.8 g/kg/day (0.36 g/lb/day).
- Vegetable protein should be considered an alternative to animal protein.

Is it beneficial to consume omega-3 fatty acids? What foods are the best sources of omega-3?

Recent scientific research has shown that diets which are high in polyunsaturated fatty acids have effects similar to monounsaturated fatty acids on plasma lipid concentrations. More specifically, omega-3 polyunsaturated fatty acids seem to have a cardioprotective role and can lower the plasma levels of triglycerides, both of which are beneficial for people with diabetes. Therefore, almost all the diabetes associations (ADA, DNSG, DUK) advise the consumption of two to three servings of fish (preferably oily fish, not the commercially fried fish filets) each week and plant sources of omega-3 fatty acids (e.g. rapeseed oil, soybean oil, nuts and some green leafy vegetables). The most common food sources of omega-3 are mackerel, salmon, sardines, pilchards, sild, fresh tuna, halibut and shrimp, tofu, scallops, snapper flaxseeds, walnuts, rapeseed oil and soybeans.

Are phytosterols useful for diabetic subjects?

Plant sterols and plant stanols, which are known as 'phytosterols', are plant compounds with a chemical structure very similar to that of cholesterol. Thus, plant sterol and stanol esters can be used to block the intestinal absorption of both dietary and biliary cholesterol and to decrease the amount of cholesterol absorbed into the bloodstream. By lowering both total and low-density lipoprotein (LDL) cholesterol levels, phytosterols may play a crucial dietary role in reducing the risk of heart disease. At the same time, recent research has shown that some types of phytosterols (beta-sitosterol, beta-sistosterolin) can stimulate, to a certain extent, insulin secretion and may improve blood glucose control, excluding the regulation of cholesterol. One possible mechanism is through the effect of sterols (e.g. beta-sitosterol) on the stimulation of insulin release in the presence of non-stimulatory glucose concentrations, and the inhibition of glucose-6-phosphatase.

Therefore, phytosterols could be useful for individuals with diabetes, in the sense that they can protect against atherosclerosis. It is generally suggested

Chapter 5

that a median intake of ∼2 g/day of plant sterols and stanols can contribute to the lowering of the plasma total and LDL cholesterol. Regular food sources of sterols are rice bran, wheat germ, different types of corn oils and soybeans. In addition, a wide range of functional foods and beverages (e.g. margarine, spreads and salad dressing, milk and yoghurt) are available from the food industry, products that are good sources of both plant sterols and stanols. These products should be used cautiously and not simply added to the diet in order to avoid weight gain. It is also noted that phytosterols can be found in the human body only at very low levels, as they are hard to absorb.

Are trans fatty acids harmful to diabetic subjects?

Trans fat is a type of unsaturated fat, with a trans-isomer fatty acid(s) configuration, which can be either monounsaturated or polyunsaturated. Trans fats are naturally present in foods, but they are mainly industrially created by hydrogenating or partially hydrogenating plant oils in the presence of a catalyst, a process which was developed in the early 1900s. They are produced and used in the food industry, mainly because they have a higher melting point and a longer shelf-life. Food products which are high trans fatty acid (TFA) sources are pastry foods such as pasties and pork pies, some processed food products, stock cubes, French fries, microwave oven popcorn, chocolate bars, some types of crisps, biscuits and fast food. Trans fatty acids, such as conjugated linoleic acid and vaccenic acid, naturally occur, at a level of 2–5%, in the milk and body fat of ruminants (cows and sheep). This specific type of fat is neither required nor beneficial for health. In general, trans fats have been shown to raise LDL cholesterol (even more that saturated fatty acids) and lower high-density lipoprotein (HDL) cholesterol. Their contribution to the risk of ischaemic heart disease (IHD) has recently gained further support, following the results of large, prospective population-based studies. When compared to saturated fat, TFAs are associated with a considerably (from 2.5 to more than 10-fold sometimes) higher risk increment for IHD. Health authorities recommend that the consumption of trans fat should be reduced to small or even trace amounts. World health and diabetes associations such as the American Diabetes Association recommend that the intake of trans unsaturated fatty acids should be minimised by people with diabetes, while the Diabetes and Nutrition Study Group (DNSG) recommends that the combination of saturated fats and TFAs should be lower than 10%, or sometimes lower than 8%, in individuals with elevated LDL-cholesterol. Recent evidence that there is no safe level for the intake of artificially created trans fats is growing.

Can the overconsumption of olive oil be harmful to people with diabetes?

The primary dietary goal for people with diabetes is to limit saturated, TFA and cholesterol intake and to increase the intake of monounsaturated and omega-3 fatty acids to reduce the risk of cardiovascular disease. The consumption of olive oil lowers the risk of heart disease by increasing HDL cholesterol and lowering LDL cholesterol. Substituting olive oil, which is a monounsaturated fat, for saturated fat in the diet will help a person's heart and general health condition and fat mass loss, and at lower triglyceride levels. Various studies of diabetic patients have shown that meals containing olive oil lower blood sugar levels better than meals that are low in fat do. A daily moderate amount of olive oil can protect from oxidative stress (free radical damage to cholesterol), whereas a higher consumption does not. This means that consuming more than a couple of tablespoons at a meal can increase free radical damage of cholesterol and at the same time will increase the caloric intake, which will lead to body weight gain and the development of obesity.

What are the recommendations for alcohol intake for people with diabetes?

The recommendations for alcohol intake are almost the same as for the general population. A large number of prospective population studies in the past decade, and in many countries, have shown a J-shaped association between alcohol intake and mortality, reporting a beneficial effect in light-to-moderate and a detrimental effect in high alcohol consumption. A sensible alcohol intake of ≤2 standard drinks or alcohol units per day and more specifically <14 standard drinks per week for men and <9 for women, consumed always with food to avoid mainly nocturnal hypoglycaemia, is the general advice for people with diabetes. Moderate alcohol consumption of this level may have a cardioprotective effect, reducing the risk of cardiovascular disease. If individuals choose to drink alcohol, their daily intake should be limited to the above quantities. Thus, alcohol intake is a significant predictor of coronary events and a low-to-moderate intake seems to be associated with a reduction in the prevalence of acute coronary events (ACEs) in diabetes, whereas higher consumption is associated with an increase in lipids and blood pressure levels, and in the risk of developing ACEs. In certain cases, such as women in pregnancy, people with a history of alcoholism and those with medical problems (e.g. pancreatitis, liver disease, severe hypertriglyceridaemia and neuropathy), abstention from alcohol should be advised.

What types of alcohol should diabetic people consume?

Diabetic subjects should be aware not only of the total quantity of alcohol and timing of consumption in moderate quantities but also of the type of alcohol consumed. Red wine, medium-dry white wine, light beer (lager), whisky, gin and vodka, combined or mixed with diet soft drinks, diet tonic, club soda, seltzer or water can be consumed, always with meals or after having a meal. On the other hand, sweet wine, port wine, any form of darkened beer, cocktails, mixed spirits and liquors, mix drinks with tonic, which have a high sugar

Chapter 5

content, should be avoided. It is important to note that alcoholic drinks must be consumed with meals or after having a meal, since alcohol is by itself a hypoglycaemic factor.

Does alcohol intake have any effect on triglycerides?

Excessive alcohol intake and elevated glucose concentrations are often reported to be the cause of secondary hypertriglyceridaemia. People with diabetes and hypertriglyceridaemia are often advised to avoid alcoholic beverages, especially in the case of hypertriglyceridaemic diabetic subjects. According to the general recommendations of diabetic associations (ADA, BDA, DNSG), abstention from alcohol should be advised for people with severe hypertriglyceridaemia, as elevated triglyceride levels are assumed to be a risk factor for cardiovascular disease. At the same time, recent observational, epidemiological studies, and meta-analyses of these studies, conducted on diabetic persons without hypertriglyceridaemia show that the limited intake of less than one drink per day for adult women and less than two drinks per day for adult men has little or even no association between alcohol intake and triglyceride levels, while they show a general benefit, of alcohol consumption, on cardiovascular risk in patients with diabetes. In these studies, one beverage containing alcohol is defined as 350 ml (12.25 fl oz) of beer, 150 ml (5.25 fl oz) of wine or 40 ml (1.4 fl oz) of distilled spirits; any of these contain approximately 15 g of alcohol (ethanol).

Is it necessary for diabetic subjects to take multivitamin supplements?

It is generally accepted that people with diabetes, type 1 or 2, should meet their nutritional needs by consuming a well-balanced diet, based on the guidelines of diabetes associations and organisations. It is also accepted that vitamin and mineral supplementation is not generally recommended, unless there is a certain identified deficiency or need, or a limited dietary intake of a specific nutrient or group of foods (e.g. limited intake of fruits and vegetables or dairy products). As the latest evidence suggests that the levels of free radicals are higher in people with diabetes and that diabetes is a state of increased oxidative stress, an antioxidant supplementation (vitamin C and E or beta-carotene in certain doses) could be discussed with people with diabetes, especially with smokers. At the same time, it is evidence based by different studies that beta-carotene supplements, in high doses, increase the risk of lung cancer, especially in smokers.

It must be made clear that any dietary supplement should be given only under the advice of a doctor or clinical dietitian, as there is evidence that long-term supplementation could be harmful, and even toxic. Thus, megadoses of certain antioxidants, such as vitamin E and C, beta-carotene and selenium, do not have a protective action against heart diseases or forms of cancer, but they could lead to toxic reactions and other health problems.

Which micronutrients are necessary for the diet of a child or adult with diabetes?

It is generally accepted that there is no clear benefit from vitamin and mineral supplementation for subjects with diabetes. Only in the case of uncontrolled diabetes may it be necessary to provide vitamin and mineral supplementation in order to avoid or to treat micronutrient deficiency. Diabetic subjects should meet their daily mineral and vitamin needs by eating a healthy diet, including fresh food sources from all the food groups. All micronutrients are necessary for both the adult and child with diabetes in order to achieve a good state of health, and good glycaemic control. Antioxidant substances (vitamin A, C, E, selenium), chromium, magnesium and zinc seem to have a beneficial effect on protecting the subject with diabetes from oxidative stress, on glucose control and on carbohydrate intolerance, but only when absorbed from foods.

What are the sodium/salt allowances?

It is widely accepted that a modest reduction in the intake of dietary salt (sodium chloride) can improve blood pressure and proteinuria in patients with hypertension. For people with diabetes, in the presence of hypertension, a reduced sodium intake at a level ranging from 4.6 g/day to 2.3 g/day is advised or up to 6 g of sodium chloride (salt) per day. For people with diabetes and severe hypertension or nephropathy, sodium intake should be even lower (<2,000 mg/day). In order to achieve this reduction, it is suggested not only to avoid salt use in cooking or at the table but also to avoid salt-rich foods (e.g. processed meats, canned foods, sauces, pickles) and instead to eat salt-free bread and crisps and to choose fresh or frozen meats and vegetables.

Chapter 5

When is it necessary to use carbohydrate counting?

Carbohydrate counting can help insulin-dependent individuals and people with type 1 diabetes in achieving better blood glucose control, while providing considerable variety in their diet. Carbohydrate counting can be used in meal-planning strategies that allow for both consistent and inconsistent carbohydrate intake (i.e. with insulin/carbohydrate ratios). In the Diabetes Control and Complications Trial, participants with a consistent carbohydrate intake generally found it easier to reach target blood glucose than those who ate carbohydrate inconsistently did. However, since the focus is on carbohydrate, care must be taken to help people with diabetes achieve a nutritionally adequate diet.

What type of physical activity is suitable for diabetic subjects?

Physical activity is considered a cornerstone of the medical management of diabetes, alongside a proper diet and medications/insulin, when compulsory.

A recent review by the ADA suggests that all types of activity can, under the appropriate circumstances, be beneficial for diabetic people. Structured exercise, aerobic fitness or resistant training are all important, especially for type 2 diabetes. Structured exercise, which has an increased intensity, has a positive effect on glycaemic control. Physical activity, through aerobic exercise, contributes to decreasing cardiovascular and overall mortality and increasing levels of HDL. Finally, resistance training is also beneficial, as it improves insulin sensitivity and has a positive effect on reduced muscle mass, although increased care should be taken to ensure it is performed safely. The patient's condition should be evaluated before any type of physical activity is suggested. This is appropriate for all people with diabetes. Age, weight and BMI, previous activity level, type of therapy and risk of cardiovascular or coronary artery disease are some of the factors that should be investigated before suggesting one type of activity. Physical activity can help the general health of a diabetic person, even without dramatic changes in body fat and total weight, simply by reducing their insulin resistance and increasing their insulin sensitivity.

Is it necessary to exercise daily in order to lose weight?

The combination of diet, behaviour modification and exercise/physical activity seems to be the best way to achieve long-term weight control for people with diabetes, and especially those with type 2. The adoption of a better way of eating according to dietary recommendations, exercising and being more active and leading a generally healthy lifestyle can drastically help the diabetic person to achieve an ideal weight and BMI, and to decrease cardiovascular risk. The World Health Organization (WHO) suggests 60–90 minutes of moderate physical activity a day in order to lose weight by exercise alone (without dietary modification). By achieving the goal of 10,000 steps/day (equivalent to 30 min of daily activity) or having approximately seven hours of moderate to vigorous exercise per week, the diabetic person will succeed in maintaining a long-term maintenance of their achieved weight loss.

Physical activity or diet? Is the combination of both better than only one of them?

The combination of diet, behaviour modification and exercise/physical activity is important and necessary, not only for weight loss and maintenance but also for better glucose control. This means that it is difficult to lose weight and to attain sufficient blood glucose control if one chooses to either follow a low-fat, low-calorie diet while being totally inactive or exercise while overeating. The above combination is essential for minimising lean body mass loss and decreasing the waist-to-hip ratio. Physical activity, when used in combination with a calorie-restricted diet in overweight individuals, is also important for the improvement of coronary heart health and the increase of the resting metabolic rate and HDL.

Is it necessary to match different types of insulin to a proper diet?

The type of diet and the time plan of meals depend on the type of insulin the diabetic person takes. There are different types of insulin, such as basal, rapid, short, intermediate and, finally, long-acting, which are taken in simple injections or in premixed combinations. Each of them acts in a different way and demands a different way of eating. Thus, a rapid-acting insulin is taken 15 min before, or even just before, eating, while a short-acting (regular) insulin is taken 30 min before meals, and a long-acting basal insulin is taken once a day at bedtime or twice, without any match with the meals, as it is usually combined with rapid-acting insulin, which is taken with the meals.

Is there a perfect or ideal meal pattern for diabetic subjects?

In diabetic subjects, the meal pattern plays a crucial role in blood glucose control. In most cases, it is essential to divide the total food and carbohydrate intake into as many meals and snacks as possible and to provide a plan compatible with the patient's lifestyle, work timetable (e.g. shift work) and method of treatment in order to achieve the best control of their diabetes. The meal plan and the number of snacks and meals in people with diabetes on medications are different from those taking insulin. Usually, diabetic subjects taking insulin are advised to space their meals in order to cover the peaks and basal effects of insulin, hence they need to receive a mid-morning, a mid-afternoon and a bedtime snack so as to diminish the gap between two main meals and to avoid hypoglycaemia. Therefore, there is no ideal meal pattern and both the number of meals eaten each day and the time at which the meals are eaten each day vary from person to person. Thus, every diabetic subject should consult a physician or a clinical dietitian for proper guidance.

What factors influence the recommended meal pattern for a diabetic person?

Various factors can influence the meal pattern of a diabetic subject. The total nutritional and energy requirements, the type of pharmacological treatment (medications or insulin, either long or short acting), blood glucose measurements, the presence of frequent hypo- or hyperglycaemias, the level, the frequency and the duration of physical activity and the body weight of the diabetic subject are the most important factors that should be taken into consideration by the dietitian before proposing the appropriate meal plan.

What types of in-between snacks can a diabetic subject consume?

In many cases, people with diabetes on insulin are advised to consume in-between snacks in order to avoid hypoglycaemia and to improve their glucose control. Some of the snacks suggested are a piece of fruit, a bowl of milk and low-fat and sugar-free cereals, cheese and crackers, low-fat or sugar-free yogurt, a bowl of soup, a cereal bar, digestive or other low-sugar biscuits, melba toast with low-fat margarine, salt-free nuts or almonds. All of these snacks provide mainly carbohydrates, with protein or fat, and help diabetic people to keep their blood glucose levels steady between their main meals.

How can we treat hypoglycaemia with diet? What are the most appropriate foods?

'Hypoglycaemia' is the term for a blood glucose level lower than normal or for the dropping from a high blood glucose level to a normal one very quickly. Hypoglycaemia can occur from certain dietary or pharmacological mistakes or certain illnesses, such as liver disease and some types of tumour. As far as concerns the severity of the condition, it can be categorised as:

- mild, when autonomic symptoms (usually sweating, palpitations, trembling) are present and patients are able to treat themselves
- moderate, when autonomic and neuroglycopaenic symptoms are present and they are able to treat themselves
- severe, when the affected person requires assistance of another person, there is unconsciousness and the plasma glucose level is often below 2.8 mmol/l (52 mg/dl).

In order to treat the hypoglycaemia, we should provide easily absorbed carbohydrates and mainly glucose, which will produce an increase in blood glucose in safe levels and relieve symptoms. Foods or food elements appropriate for the treatment of hypoglycaemia are:

- 15–20 g of glucose (three glucose tablets)
- a piece of white bread
- 1 tablespoon of table sugar (dissolved in water)
- $^1/_2$ cup of juice or regular soft drink
- 1 tablespoon of honey or corn syrup or two tablespoons of jam
- $^1/_2$ cup of fat-free milk
- $^1/_2$ tube of glucose gel (quite slowly absorbed, should be swallowed with fluids).

Glucose is preferable since it is quickly absorbed. It is also noted that for those persons who are unconscious glucagon injections, administered by another person are indicated, unless glucose can be administered by a doctor or a nurse via an IV. If the person does not have a main meal within an hour, an extra snack containing carbohydrates should be advised.

How do we support a child with type 2 diabetes nutritionally?

As already mentioned for individuals with type 2 diabetes, impaired glucose tolerance or impaired fasting glucose, attention to food portions and weight management combined with physical activity are the key points for good glycaemic control. The main cause of the development of type 2 diabetes in children is overweight and obesity. So, the fundamental goal in the nutritional treatment of this type of diabetes is to combine weight loss with a well-balanced diet to normalise blood glucose and glycated haemoglobin (HbA1c) and thereby decrease the risk of acute and chronic diabetic complications. The level of calorie restriction depends on the severity of obesity, the age and the level of activity. The child with type 2 diabetes should follow an active lifestyle, avoid frequent snacking on energy-dense foods, have frequent meals with a good amount of fibre and high biological value protein as well as low-fat foods. They should also aim to reduce their intake of simple sugars.

Gestational diabetes

How many kcal should we provide to a woman with gestational diabetes?

Gestational diabetes, also known as 'gestational diabetes mellitus' (GDM) or 'diabetes during pregnancy', is a type of diabetes that is diagnosed in the course of a pregnancy. The aims of the dietary therapy in gestational diabetes are the provision of:

- adequate maternal and foetal nutrition
- energy intake for appropriate weight gain
- adequate protein intake
- any necessary micronutrients (vitamins and minerals).

When, at the beginning of pregnancy, the body weight is normal, energy needs are not significantly increased in the first trimester, while an additional 300–350 kcal/day (1256–1465 kJ/day) are suggested during the second and third trimesters. This extra energy is required for certain procedures, such as the increase of the maternal blood volume and of the amniotic fluids, the increase of the breast and other tissues, placental and foetal growth.

The amount of calories (and carbohydrate and other nutrients) that will be needed depends on several factors, such as the woman's weight before pregnancy, her current weight gain, her current physical activity level and her blood glucose levels. Energy intake should ensure a desirable weight gain during pregnancy, as it is important to avoid any excessive weight gain. A minimum energy intake per day must not be lower than 1700–1800 kcal (7118–7536 kJ), and these calories should come from foods of a high nutritious value. A well-balanced dietary plan is important from the beginning of the pregnancy in order to avoid excess body weight intake and obesity and reduce the danger of macrosomic babies. It is generally recommended to avoid hypocaloric diets, mainly in obese women with gestational diabetes, because these can result in ketonaemia and ketonuria.

Chapter 5

Do we decrease the amount of carbohydrate in the diet in gestational diabetes?

Nutritional requirements during pregnancy and lactation are similar for women with and without diabetes. In both cases, the percentage of energy derived from carbohydrates should be 45–55%, mostly from complex carbohydrates and less from simple carbohydrates and sugars. Nutritional therapy for gestational diabetes should focus mainly on the appropriate number and plan of meals, the right food choices for appropriate weight gain, normoglycaemia and finally the absence of ketones. The diabetic pregnant woman is advised to use the carbohydrate (bread) exchange system, to consume a lot of vegetables and fruits, whole wheat products and to avoid sweets and other sugary foods. In cases of gestational diabetes, where it is difficult or even impossible to achieve good glucose control, through diet and medications, a modest carbohydrate restriction, from all the meals, may be appropriate, according to the specific needs of the pregnant woman.

More often, in cases where the morning levels of glucose are high, owing to increased levels of growth hormone and cortisol (the so-called dawn phenomenon), a modest carbohydrate restriction, from 15 to 45 g, from breakfast is necessary, in order to help the pregnant woman tolerate the carbohydrates.

How much protein can we provide to a woman with gestational diabetes?

As mentioned above, the nutritional requirements, during pregnancy, remain the same for women with and without diabetes. As far as concerns their protein intake, pregnant diabetic women need to consume adequate protein every day – 0.75 g/kg/day (0.34 g/lb/day) – plus an additional 10 g/day or 15–20% of total energy intake, mostly from low-fat animal sources such as meat, dairy products, egg, fish, poultry, and from legumes and starchy foods.

Diabetes and renal disease

How much protein should we provide to a diabetic person with nephropathy?

The most recent recommendations for protein intake in diabetic nephropathy suggest approximately a recommended dietary allowance (RDA) for an adult of 0.8 g/kg/day (0.36 g/lb/day) (~10% of daily energy intake). A dietary intake of protein at this level has been associated with the reduction of albuminuria and the stabilisation of kidney function and is estimated and based on an idealised body weight, to avoid the overestimation of dietary protein intake.

Chapter 5

However, in cases where the glomerular filtration rate (GFR) begins to fall, a further restriction to 0.6 g/kg/day (0.27 g/lb/day) may be useful in slowing the decline of GFR in selected patients. It is crucial to design the dietary plan of the person with diabetes in such a way as to avoid nutritional deficiency, which can be associated with muscle weakness. However, nutritional studies indicate that most patients do not easily comply with these restrictions.

Should we provide more carbohydrates to patients with diabetic nephropathy?

Considering that dietary protein intake should be limited in patients with diabetic nephropathy, an increased intake of carbohydrate (and/or fats) is required in order to achieve an adequate energy intake. The total non-protein calories make up approximately 90% of the total caloric intake, 60% of which should be from carbohydrates and the rest, 30% or less, from fats. This high amount of carbohydrates must be derived mainly from whole grains, fruits and vegetables, which should be carefully chosen, in order to not disturb the levels of sodium, potassium and phosphorus in the body.

What type of fruit and vegetable should we include in the diet of a person with diabetic nephropathy?

In diabetic nephropathy, owing to kidney function decline, there is a parallel weakening of the kidney's ability to filter potassium. Thus, it is essential to avoid a consequent rise in serum potassium, by reducing the consumption of potassium-rich foods such as fruits and fruit juices, some vegetables and chocolate. This rise could lead to cardiac arrhythmias or even cardiac arrest. When a diabetic subject is at the pre-end-stage renal disease (ESRD), dietary potassium is usually restricted whenever serum potassium levels are higher than normal. Individuals on haemodialysis need to follow a potassium-restricted diet, while on peritoneal dialysis, owing to frequent filtration, they will usually need to supplement high-potassium foods as their serum potassium may be low. Higher levels of potassium may occur also because of some hypertension medications.

Common high-potassium foods, which may need to be restricted, are fruit juices, apricot, banana, orange, kiwi, mango, dried fruits, asparagus, avocado, potato (although potatoes can be boiled in lots of water in order to reduce their potassium content), tomato, wild rice, wholegrain rice and pasta, nuts and seed, legumes, coconut and chocolate. Common low-potassium foods, which may be consumed in moderation, are apple, pear, peach, pineapple, clementine, broccoli, cabbage, cucumber, eggplant, peppers, green beans, white rice, cornflakes, rice cereals, white pasta, noodles and spices. Low-sodium products, such as Lo Salt, contain potassium chloride and should be avoided.

Further reading

AACE Diabetes Mellitus Clinical Practice Guidelines Task Force (2007) American Association of Clinical Endocrinologists Medical Guidelines for Clinical Practice for the Management of Diabetes Mellitus. *Endocrine Practice* **13**(suppl. 1), http://www.aace.com/pub/pdf/guidelines/DMGuidelines2007.pdf, [accessed 10th February 2010].

American Diabetes Association (2003) Implications of the Diabetes Control and Complications Trial. *Diabetes Care* **26**(suppl.): S25–7.

American Diabetes Association, Bantle JP, Wylie-Rosett J *et al.* (2008) Nutrition recommendations and interventions for diabetes: A position statement of the American Diabetes Association. *Diabetes Care* **31**(suppl. 1): S61–78.

Bantle JP, Beebe CA, Brunzell JD *et al.* (2002) Evidence-based nutrition principles and recommendations for the treatment and prevention of diabetes and related complications. *Diabetes Care* **25**: 148–98.

Brand-Miller J, Hayne S, Petocz P, Colagiuri S (2003) Low-glycemic index diets in the management of diabetes: A meta-analysis of randomized controlled trials. *Diabetes Care* **26**: 2261–7.

Department of Health and Human Services/Department of Agriculture (2005) *Dietary Guidelines for Americans.* US Government Printing Office, Washington.

Diabetes Prevention Program Research Group (2002) Reduction in the incidence of type 2 diabetes with lifestyle intervention or metformin. *New England Journal of Medicine* **346**: 393–403.

Katsilambros N, Diakoumopoulou E, Ioannidis I *et al.* (2006) *Diabetes in Clinical Practice: Questions and answers from case studies.* John Wiley & Sons, Ltd, Chichester.

Katsilambros N, Kostas G, Michalakis N *et al.* (1997) Metabolic effects of long-term diets enriched in olive oil or sunflower oil in non-insulin-dependent diabetes. *Nutrition, Metabolism, and Cardiovascular Diseases* **6**: 164–7.

Kidney Disease Outcomes Quality Initiative (2007) Clinical practice guidelines and clinical practice recommendations for diabetes and chronic kidney disease. *American Journal of Kidney Diseases* **49**(2, suppl. 2): S12–154.

Klein S, Sheard NF, Pi-Sunyer X *et al.* (2004) Weight management through lifestyle modification for the prevention and management of type 2 diabetes: Rationale and strategies: A statement of the American Diabetes Association, the North American Association for the Study of Obesity, and the American Society for Clinical Nutrition. *Diabetes Care* **27**: 2067–73.

Krauss RM, Eckel RH, Howard B *et al.* (2000). AHA Dietary Guidelines: Revision 2000: A statement for healthcare professionals from the Nutrition Committee of the American Heart Association. *Circulation* **102**: 2284–99.

Mann JI, De Leeuw I, Hermansen K *et al.* (2004) Evidence-based nutritional approaches to the treatment and prevention of diabetes mellitus. *Nutrition, Metabolism, and Cardiovascular Diseases* **14**: 373–94.

Nutrition Subcommittee of the Diabetes Care Advisory Committee of Diabetes UK (2003) The implementation of nutritional advice for people with diabetes. *Diabetic Medicine* **20**: 786–807.

O'Keefe JH, Gheewala NM, O'Keefe JO (2008) Dietary strategies for improving postprandial glucose, lipids, inflammation, and cardiovascular health. *Journal of the American College of Cardiology* **51**(3): 249–55.

Pitsavos C, Makrilakis K, Panagiotakos DB *et al.* (2005) The J-shape effect of alcohol intake on the risk of developing acute coronary syndromes in diabetic subjects: the CARDIO2000 II Study. *Diabetic Medicine* **22**(3): 243–8.

Sigal RJ, Kenny GP, Wasserman DH, Castaneda-Sceppa C (2004) Physical activity/exercise and type 2 diabetes. *Diabetes Care* **27**: 2518–39.

Sigal RJ, Kenny GP, Wasserman DH *et al.* (2006) Physical activity/exercise and type 2 diabetes: A consensus statement from the American Diabetes Association. *Diabetes Care* **29**: 1433–8.

Trichopoulou A, Orfanos P, Norat T *et al.* (2005) Modified Mediterranean diet and survival: EPIC elderly prospective cohort study. *British Medical Journal* **330**(7498): 991.

US Renal Data System (2005) *Annual Data Report.* The National Institutes of Health, National Institute of Diabetes and Digestive and Kidney Diseases, Bethesda, MD.

Wang C, Harris WS, Chung M *et al.* (2006) n-3 Fatty acids from fish or fish-oil supplements, but not alpha-linolenic acid, benefit cardiovascular outcomes in primary- and secondary-prevention studies: A systematic review. *American Journal of Clinical Nutrition* **84**(1): 5–17.

West SG, Hecker KD, Mustad VA *et al.* (2005) Acute effects of monounsaturated fatty acids with and without omega-3 fatty acids on vascular reactivity in individuals with type 2 diabetes. *Diabetologia* **48**(1): 113–22.

Chapter 5

Chapter 6

Hypertension and Cardiovascular Diseases

Meropi Kontogianni

What are the definitions and classification of blood pressure levels?

Historically, more emphasis was placed on diastolic than on systolic blood pressure (BP) as a predictor of cardiovascular morbidity and fatal events. However, a large number of observational studies have demonstrated that cardiovascular morbidity and mortality bear a continuous relationship with both systolic and diastolic BP (Table 6.1).

Is there any relationship between body weight and blood pressure?

A substantial body of evidence from observational studies documents that body weight is directly associated with BP and that excess body fat predisposes to increased BP and hypertension. It has been estimated that 60% of hypertensives are obese and that approximately 20–30% of hypertension prevalence can be attributed to obesity. There is also conclusive evidence that weight reduction lowers BP in obese patients and has beneficial effects on associated risk factors such as insulin resistance, diabetes, hyperlipidaemia, left ventricular hypertrophy and obstructive sleep apnoea. In a meta-analysis of available studies, the mean systolic and diastolic BP reductions associated with an average weight loss of 5.1 kg were 4.4 and 3.6 mmHg, respectively. Modest weight loss, with or without sodium reduction, can prevent hypertension in overweight individuals with high normal BP and can facilitate medication step-down and drug withdrawal. Because in middle-aged individuals body weight frequently shows a progressive increase (0.5–1.5 kg per year), weight stabilisation may also be considered a useful goal to pursue.

Table 6.1 Definitions and classification of blood pressure levels (mmHg).

Category	Systolic		Diastolic
Optimal	<120	and	<80
Normal	120–129	and/or	80–84
High normal	130–139	and/or	85–89
Grade 1 hypertension	140–159	and/or	90–99
Grade 2 hypertension	160–179	and/or	100–109
Grade 3 hypertension	≥180	and/or	≥110
Isolated systolic hypertension	≥140	and	<90

Isolated systolic hypertension should be graded (1, 2, 3) according to systolic BP values in the ranges indicated, if diastolic values are <90 mmHg. Grades 1, 2 and 3 correspond to the classification of mild, moderate and severe hypertension, respectively. These terms have now been omitted to avoid confusion with quantification of total cardiovascular risk.

What is the recommended dietary approach to the prevention and treatment of hypertension?

The dietary approach to the prevention and treatment of hypertension is an integral part of the lifestyle changes that are required to control BP. The lifestyle measures that are widely agreed to lower BP or cardiovascular risk, and that should be considered in all patients are:

- smoking cessation
- weight reduction in the overweight or weight stabilisation
- moderation of alcohol consumption
- physical activity
- healthy dietary choices, which include:
  o reduction of salt intake
  o increase in potassium intake through increase in fruit and vegetable consumption
  o decrease in saturated and total fat intake.

There is also evidence that increased salt intake during childhood may result in an increased probability of hypertension during adult life.

Moreover, adherence to the Dietary Approach to Stop Hypertension (DASH) diet seems to exert a protective effect against BP and can reduce systolic BP by 8–14 mmHg. The DASH eating plan focuses on increasing the intake of foods rich in nutrients that are expected to lower BP, mainly minerals (like potassium, calcium and magnesium), protein and fibre and follows guidelines to promote a healthy heart by limiting the intake of saturated fat and cholesterol. It also includes nutrient-rich foods so that it meets other nutrient requirements as recommended by the Institute of Medicine. The DASH diet – which is high in fruits, vegetables, nuts and low-fat dairy products, emphasises an intake of fish and chicken rather than of red meat and is low in saturated fat, cholesterol, sugar and refined carbohydrate – has been shown in large randomised controlled trials to reduce BP significantly both in hypertensives and in prehypertension stage. Moreover, studies have found that the DASH menus containing 2300 mg of sodium can lower BP and that an even

Table 6.2 Food groups' distribution for a DASH dietary plan of 2000 kcal.

Food group	Number of daily servings for a 2000 kcal diet
Grains	**6–8** (1 slice bread, $^1/_2$ cup cooked rice, pasta, or cereal)
Vegetables	**4–5** (1 cup raw leafy vegetable, $^1/_2$ cup cooked vegetable)
Fruits	**4–5** (1 medium fruit, $^1/_2$ cup fruit juice)
Fat-free or low-fat milk and dairy products	**2–3** (1 cup milk or yogurt, 1.5 oz cheese)
Lean meats, poultry and fish	**≤6** (1 oz cooked meats, poultry or fish, 1 egg)
Nuts, seeds and legumes	**4–5/week** ($^1/_3$ cup or 1.5 oz nuts, $^1/_2$ cup cooked legumes)
Fats and oils	**2–3** (1 tsp soft margarine or vegetable oil)
Sweets and added sugars	**≤5/week** (1 tbsp sugar, jelly or jam)

lower level of sodium, 1500 mg, can further reduce BP. Table 6.2 describes the distribution of food groups for a DASH dietary plan of 2000 kcal.

In addition, evidence from large epidemiological studies (EPIC, SUN, ATTICA) supports the view that adherence to the Mediterranean diet (MD) can protect against high BP. In the EPIC study, the MD score was significantly inversely associated with both systolic and diastolic BP, with olive oil, vegetables and fruit being the principal factors behind the overall effect of the MD on arterial BP. According to the ATTICA study, adherence to the MD was associated with a 26% lower risk of being hypertensive and with a 36% greater probability of controlling BP.

How much salt (and sodium) should a hypertensive patient consume?

Epidemiological studies suggest that dietary salt intake is a contributor to BP elevation and to the prevalence of hypertension. Restriction of sodium intake to 2 g per day lowers systolic pressure, on average, by 3.7–4.8 mmHg and lowers diastolic pressure, on average, by 0.9–2.5 mmHg, although the reductions vary from person to person beyond these ranges. Randomised controlled trials in hypertensive patients indicate that reducing sodium intake by 80–100 mmol (4.7–5.8 g of sodium chloride) per day from an initial intake of around 180 mmol (10.5 g of sodium chloride) per day reduces BP by an average of 4–6 mmHg, although the trials also showed a great degree of variation between patients. Salt sensitivity is common in older patients with hypertension. Despite concern that salt restriction for all patients with hypertension may have adverse consequences, moderate sodium restriction appears to be generally safe and effective and particularly so in older people. The recommended adequate daily sodium intake has been recently reduced from 100 to 65 mmol/day, corresponding to 3.8 g/day of sodium chloride, which may be currently difficult to achieve. An achievable recommendation is less than 5 g/day sodium chloride (85 mmol of sodium/day).

What effect does the consumption of caffeinated coffee and alcohol have on hypertension?

The high intake of caffeinated coffee may influence BP or the risk of coronary heart disease. A single dose of caffeine of 200–250 mg, equivalent to 2–3 cups of coffee, has been shown to increase systolic BP by 3–14 mmHg and diastolic BP by 4–13 mmHg shortly after intake in normotensive subjects. However, the cardiovascular system may develop tolerance to caffeine. The objective of a meta-analysis was to quantify the chronic effect (≥ 7 days) of regular coffee and caffeine intake on BP, using data from randomised controlled trials. According to the results, regular caffeine intake increases BP, although the pressure effect of caffeine was only small if ingested through coffee. More research is needed on the cardiovascular effects of caffeine and caffeinated foods and beverages other than coffee, such as cola and sports drinks. In general, a habitual intake of about 400 mg of caffeine per day ($\sim$3–4 cups of coffee) does not increase the risk of hypertension, and nor does it affect BP control.

Many studies have shown a U- or J-shaped association of mortality with alcohol consumption, in which light and moderate drinking results in a reduced mortality compared with non-drinkers, while heavy drinkers have a rising death rate. However, some population studies indicate that the relationship between alcohol consumption, BP levels and the prevalence of hypertension is linear in populations. Beyond that, high levels of alcohol consumption are associated with a high risk of stroke; this is particularly so for binge drinking. Alcohol attenuates the effects of antihypertensive drug therapy, but this effect is at least partially reversible within 1–2 weeks by moderating one's drinking. Trials of alcohol reduction have shown a significant reduction in systolic and diastolic BP. Hypertensive patients who drink alcohol should be advised to limit their consumption to no more than 20–30 g ethanol per day for men, and hypertensive women to no more than 10–20 g ethanol per day and they should be warned against the increased risk of stroke associated with binge drinking.

Do supplements of calcium, potassium or magnesium have a place in the treatment of hypertension?

Epidemiological and metabolic studies suggest that calcium, potassium and magnesium may have a role in the regulation of BP. However, results from systematic reviews and meta-analyses have reached conflicting conclusions about whether oral supplementation of these minerals can reduce BP. Moreover, a recent Cochrane Systematic Review attempted to evaluate the effects of combined mineral supplementation as a treatment for primary hypertension in adults, but it found no robust evidence that supplements of any combination of potassium, magnesium or calcium reduce mortality, morbidity or BP in adults. Evidence so far does not support the routine supplementation with calcium, potassium or magnesium in hypertensive patients.

What is the relationship between physical activity and hypertension?

A recent meta-analysis of randomised controlled trials concluded that dynamic aerobic endurance training reduces resting systolic and diastolic BP by 3.0/2.4 mmHg, respectively and daytime ambulatory BP by 3.3/3.5 mmHg, respectively. The reduction in resting BP was more pronounced in the hypertensive group (–6.9/–4.9 mmHg) than in the normotensive one (–1.9/–1.6 mmHg). Even moderate levels of exercise lowered BP, and this type of training also reduced body weight, body fat and waist circumference and increased insulin sensitivity and high-density lipoprotein (HDL) cholesterol levels. Sedentary patients should be advised to take up exercise of moderate intensity on a regular basis, e.g. 30–45 min daily. The type of exercise should primarily be an endurance-based activity (walking, jogging, swimming) supplemented by moderate resistance exercise. Intensive resistance exercise, such as heavy weight lifting, can have a marked pressor effect and should be avoided. If hypertension is poorly controlled, heavy physical exercise as well as maximal exercise testing should be discouraged or postponed until appropriate drug treatment has been instituted and BP lowered.

What are the main diet and lifestyle goals for cardiovascular disease risk reduction?

Improving diet and lifestyle is a critical component of the American Heart Association's (AHA) strategy to prevent cardiovascular disease, the leading cause of morbidity and mortality in several countries. Box 6.1 summarises the AHA 2006 diet and lifestyle goals for cardiovascular disease risk reduction.

Box 6.1 The AHA 2006 diet and lifestyle goals for cardiovascular disease risk reduction.

- Consume an overall healthy diet.
- Aim for a healthy body weight.
- Aim for recommended levels of low-density lipoprotein (LDL) cholesterol, high-density lipoprotein (HDL) cholesterol and triglycerides.
- Aim for a normal BP.
- Aim for a normal blood glucose level.
- Be physically active.
- Avoid use of and exposure to tobacco products.

Chapter 6

What dietary and lifestyle modifications would reduce the risk of cardiovascular disease?

The AHA has composed certain guidelines for the achievement of the above-mentioned goals for the reduction of cardiovascular disease risk, as follows:

- Balance calorie intake and physical activity to achieve or maintain a healthy body weight.
- Consume a diet rich in vegetables and fruits.
- Choose wholegrain, high-fibre foods.
- Consume fish, especially oily fish, at least twice a week.
- Limit the intake of saturated fat to <7% of energy, trans fat to <1% of energy and cholesterol to <300 mg per day by:
  ○ choosing lean meats and vegetable alternatives
  ○ selecting fat-free (skimmed), 1% fat and low-fat dairy products
  ○ minimising intake of partially hydrogenated fats.
- Minimise intake of beverages and foods with added sugars.
- Choose and prepare foods with little or no salt.
- If alcohol is consumed, it should be done in moderation.
- For consumption of food that is prepared outside of the home, the AHA's *Diet and Lifestyle Recommendations* should be followed.

What are the current dietary recommendations for people with hypercholesterolaemia?

The dietary management of hypercholesterolaemia, and especially elevated LDL cholesterol, is a major goal of coronary heart disease risk management. Nutritional factors that are important for primary prevention of increased LDL cholesterol levels are saturated and trans fatty acids, dietary cholesterol and excess body weight, whereas factors that reduce LDL include polyunsaturated fatty acids, viscous fibre, plant stanols/sterols, weight loss, isoflavone-containing soy protein (limited evidence) and soy protein. The principal dietary strategy for lowering LDL cholesterol levels is to replace cholesterol-raising fatty acids (i.e. saturated and trans fatty acids) with dietary carbohydrate and/or unsaturated fatty acids. Box 6.2 summarises the basic AHA recommendations for achieving a desirable lipid profile. The above therapeutic diet options (including weight loss) are expected to decrease LDL cholesterol by 20–30%.

Concerning secondary prevention, for people at high risk or who have known cardiovascular disease (e.g. coronary heart disease), the Therapeutic Lifestyle Changes (TLC) diet has been adopted. This is the next generation of the Step II diet recommended in May 2001. That was when the National Cholesterol Education Program (NCEP) released new guidelines for cholesterol management in its *Third Report of the Expert Panel on Detection, Evaluation, and Treatment of High Blood Cholesterol in Adults (Adult Treatment Panel III* (ATP III). Table 6.3 describes in detail the TLC dietary recommendations.

Box 6.2 AHA dietary recommendations for achieving desirable blood lipid profile and especially LDL cholesterol.

- Limit foods high in saturated fats
- Replace saturated fats with lower-fat foods
- Increase type of foods with unsaturated fat
- Carefully monitor intake of food high in cholesterol
- Severely limit foods containing trans fatty acids
- Increase foods rich in viscous fibre
- Increase foods containing stanol/sterol esters (special margarines, fortified orange juice, special cocoa/chocolate bars)

What are plant sterols/stanols and how do they affect blood lipid levels?

Sterols represent a group of compounds that are an essential constituent of cell membranes in animals and plants. Cholesterol is the sterol of mammalian cells, whereas multiple sterols, or phytosterols, are produced by plants. Plant sterols are very poorly absorbed by the human intestine. The specific plant sterols that are currently incorporated into foods intended to lower blood cholesterol levels are extracted from soybean oil or tall (pine tree) oil. The plant sterols currently incorporated into foods are esterified into unsaturated

Table 6.3 TLC diet in ATP III.

Nutrient	Recommended intake as percentage of total calories
Total fat[a]	25–35%
Saturated	Less than 7%
Polyunsaturated	Up to 10%
Monounsaturated	Up to 20%
Carbohydrate[b]	50–60% of total calories
Protein[c]	Approximately 15%
Cholesterol	Less than 200 mg per day
Plant stanols/sterols	2 g per day
Increased soluble fibre	10–25 g per day
Total calories	Balance energy intake and expenditure to maintain desirable body weight and prevent weight gain
Physical activity	Include enough moderate exercise to expend at least 200 kcal per day

[a] The 25–35% fat recommendation allows for increased intake of unsaturated fat in place of carbohydrates in people with metabolic syndrome or diabetes.
[b] Carbohydrate should come mainly from foods rich in complex carbohydrates. These include grains (especially whole grains), fruits and vegetables.
[c] Soy protein may be used as a replacement for some animal products.

fatty acids (creating sterol esters) to increase lipid solubility, thus allowing maximal incorporation into a limited amount of fat. Some plant sterols currently available are saturated, to form the stanol derivatives sitostanol and campestanol, which after esterification form stanol esters.

Sterol balance studies have suggested that decreased blood cholesterol levels are attributable, at least in part, to an inhibition of cholesterol absorption. This inhibition has been ascribed to a number of mechanisms, including partitioning in the micellar phase of the intestinal lumen, presence in the unstirred water layer or other mucosa barriers that may limit transmembrane transport and alteration in rates of cholesterol esterification in the intestinal wall. Generally, the inclusion of 2 g/day of plant stanols/sterols from commercially available enriched products would be expected to reduce LDL cholesterol by 6–15%.

What lifestyle changes would help people with high blood triglycerides?

Among nutrients, the major determinant of elevated triglycerides in atherogenic dyslipidaemia is dietary carbohydrate. In general, simple sugars and rapidly hydrolysed starches have a greater glyceridaemic effect than more complex carbohydrates and those consumed in conjunction with a higher intake of fibre. The recommended level of dietary fat for people with elevated triglycerides is 25–35% of calories. Within this range, complex carbohydrates and a high-fibre diet are advised to facilitate the lowering of triglycerides and to increase the levels of HDL cholesterol and the larger, more buoyant LDL particles. In addition, there is increasing evidence to support the beneficial influence of omega-3 fatty acids in the management of hypertriglyceridaemia, in doses ~3 g per day and the detrimental effect of excessive alcohol intake. Finally, for hypertriglyceridaemic people who are overweight or obese, weight loss through dietary energy restriction is the primary aim of the therapy.

Are there any dietary factors with unproven or uncertain effects on cardiovascular disease risk?

Although observational studies have suggested that high intakes of antioxidant vitamins from food and supplements are associated with a lower risk of cardiovascular disease, clinical trials of antioxidant vitamin supplements have not confirmed the benefit. Some trials, in fact, have documented potential harm, including an increased risk of lung cancer from beta-carotene supplements in smokers and an increased risk of heart failure and the possibility of increased total mortality from high-dose vitamin E supplements. Antioxidant vitamin supplements or other supplements such as selenium to prevent cardiovascular disease are not recommended. Although antioxidant supplements are not recommended, food sources of antioxidant nutrients, principally from a variety of plant-derived foods such as fruits, vegetables, whole grains and vegetable oils, are recommended.

As far as soy protein is concerned, evidence of a direct cardiovascular health benefit from consuming soy protein products instead of dairy or other proteins or of isoflavone supplements is minimal. Although earlier research has suggested that soy protein has clinically important favourable effects on LDL cholesterol levels and other cardiovascular disease risk factors, studies reported more recently have not confirmed those results. Nevertheless, consumption of foods rich in soy protein may indirectly reduce cardiovascular disease risk if they replace animal and dairy products that contain saturated fat and cholesterol.

Folate intake and to a lesser extent intake of vitamins B_6 and B_{12} are inversely associated with blood homocysteine levels. In observational studies, increased blood levels of homocysteine are associated with an increased risk of cardiovascular disease. Trials of homocysteine-reducing vitamin therapy have been disappointing, however. Available evidence is inadequate to recommend folate and other B vitamin supplements as a means to reduce cardiovascular disease risk at this time.

What is the effect of fish oils on cardiovascular disease risk? Are they indicated for the treatment of hypertension?

Fish intake has been associated with a decreased risk of cardiovascular disease. The consumption of two servings ($\approx$8 oz, $\approx$230 g) per week of fish high in 20-carbon eicosapentaenoic acid (EPA) and the 22-carbon docosahexaenoic acid (DHA) is associated with a reduced risk of both sudden death and death from coronary artery disease in adults. Patients with documented coronary heart disease are advised to consume $\approx$1 g of EPA and DHA per day, preferably from oily fish (e.g. mackerel, herrings, salmon), although EPA and DHA supplements could be considered in consultation with their physician. For individuals with hypertriglyceridaemia, 2–4 g of EPA and DHA per day, provided as capsules under a physician's care, are recommended.

Omega-3 fatty acids have also been associated with reduced BP. According to a recent systematic review of randomised controlled trials which compared fish oil supplements in supplied doses ranging from 0.1 to 17 g/day (typically about 60% eicosapentaenoic and 40% docosahexaenoic) with a placebo, both given as capsules taken several times a day, a beneficial effect on both systolic and diastolic BP was revealed in patients taking fish oil supplements. The effect of fish oils on BP is significant mainly in hypertensives and in doses of >3 g per day.

What is the best nutritional approach for the prevention and treatment of metabolic syndrome?

Metabolic syndrome is a clustering of metabolic abnormalities and cardiovascular disease risk factors (mainly visceral obesity, dyslipidaemia, hypertension and hyperglycaemia) that occur in individuals with impaired insulin resistance

Chapter 6

and subclinical inflammation. The best nutritional approach for the prevention and treatment of metabolic syndrome is based on nutrients and foods that limit insulin resistance and inflammation. Therefore, the administration of a moderate-carbohydrate, high-monounsaturated fatty acid diet seems the best approach. Carbohydrate may range from 45 to 55% of total energy intake with an emphasis on food items rich in complex carbohydrates (particularly a high content of soluble fibres) and with a low glycaemic index (GI) and restriction of simple sugars, whereas fat may range from 30 to 40% of daily energy intake with an emphasis on monounsaturated fatty acids. Moreover, a restriction of alcohol intake to <30 g per day and of salt intake to <4 g per day seems to offer additional benefit, as well as the control of body weight if the patient is overweight, through a restriction in energy intake.

Recently, epidemiological and clinical evidence support a beneficial effect of the MD in the prevention and treatment of metabolic syndrome; however, more randomised trials are needed to confirm this effect.

What dietary modifications should patients receiving warfarin tablets follow?

Warfarin is an anticoagulant agent and is used to prevent heart attacks, strokes and blood clots in veins and arteries. On the other hand, vitamin K plays a role in promoting the formation of blood clots in the body. Warfarin decreases blood clotting by acting on vitamin K. For this reason, patients receiving warfarin need to avoid sudden changes in the ingested amount of vitamin K; however, they do not need to completely avoid vitamin K. Foods that are rich in vitamin K include liver, other organ meats and green and leafy vegetables such as asparagus, parsley, collard greens, kale, dark-green lettuce, Swiss chard, turnip greens, spinach, cabbage, Brussels sprouts, broccoli, okra, scallions (green spring onions), watercress, bok choy, coriander, green beans and green peas. Stable intake of these foods every day is permitted in order to let the doctor arrange the best drug dose. Great variations in alcohol consumption should also be avoided and small amounts of daily alcohol intake or complete abstinence are recommended for people taking warfarin. Patients should be informed that cranberries and cranberry juice can interfere with warfarin kinetics and so should be completely avoided by people taking this drug. Additionally, several dietary supplements (e.g. omega-3 fatty acids, garlic, gingko biloba, ginseng, St John's wort), vitamins, minerals or herbs may interact with warfarin and should be taken only under medical and dietetic supervision.

What are the main nutritional aspects of cerebrovascular accidents/stroke management?

Nutrition has two roles concerning cerebrovascular accidents: first, to prevent them through the adoption of a healthy lifestyle, as that recommended above for cardiovascular disease risk reduction; second, to treat patients at the acute phase after the accident, as well as to alleviate problems that commonly follow a stroke, such as dysphagia.

The nutritional priorities during the acute phase of a stroke are:

- assessment of nutritional needs and nutritional status (ideally within 48 hours of admission)
- estimation of patient's ability to self-feed and swallow impairment
- coverage of nutrient and fluid needs through the appropriate route.

For a period of 4–8 weeks afterwards, the stroke patient may exhibit increased energy and protein needs, as a result of muscular atrophies. During this time, the patient should undergo a nutritional assessment, and a proper nutrition care plan should be conducted by the nutrition team. A stress factor of 5% for cerebrovascular accident and of 30% for cerebral haemorrhage should be added when estimating the basal metabolic rate. Protein needs may also increase, but generally an intake of 1–1.2 g/kg of body weight covers patient needs. Other common problems that influence the dietary regime are glucose intolerance owing to catabolic hormone effects, fluid, electrolyte or acid-base imbalances.

Respectively, the nutritional priorities in the rehabilitation phase are to:

- minimise the risk of another stroke
- help the patient resume a normal and well-balanced eating pattern, which takes into account any neurological deficits, such as dysphagia
- ensure nutrient adequacy of the diet and prevent problems of under- or overnutrition.

What is cardiac cachexia and what are the therapeutic approaches to it?

Cardiac cachexia is a common problem in patients with congestive heart failure, and its occurrence establishes a poor prognosis in patients with congestive heart failure, independently of whether the heart failure is regarded as mild or advanced. The transition from stable disease to cardiac cachexia is not well understood. Mechanisms that maintain the wasting process involve neurohormones and pro-inflammatory cytokines, which contribute to an imbalance in anabolic and catabolic pathways. A decrease in food intake alone rarely triggers the development of a wasting process, but dietary deficiencies in micronutrients and macronutrients contribute to the progression of the disease. Malabsorption from the gut as a result of bowel-wall oedema and decreased bowel perfusion also plays an important role. The therapeutic approaches to cardiac cachexia include:

- prevention of weight loss through a proper nutritional intervention
- dietary supplementation (the evidence suggests that multiple micronutrient supplementation is potentially beneficial for cachectic patients and it should contain antioxidant supplements and B-group vitamins. Food that

Chapter 6

counteracts inflammatory processes can generally be recommended, for example fish oil supplements, olives, flaxseed oil, any fruits or vegetables, garlic, ginger, turmeric, sunflower seeds, eggs, herring or nuts. Enteral nutrition should always be preferred over parenteral feeding. If parenteral nutrition becomes paramount, the general guidelines should be followed: 35 kcal/kg of body weight per day, 1.2 g of protein/kg per day, and a 70:30 glucose/lipid ratio for the non-protein energy

- pharmacotherapy (eventually, interventions with appetite stimulants, anabolic steroids and growth hormone).

What are the dietary recommendations for patients with congestive heart failure?

Although it is generally considered that a diet high in sodium is harmful (and may result in acute decompensation of congestive heart failure through a volume overload mechanism), little is known about the other aspects of diet in congestive heart failure, in terms of both general nutrition and micronutrients, such as vitamins and minerals. In congestive heart failure patients, it is important not only to properly screen for and aggressively treat the traditional risk factors of coronary heart disease (the main cause of congestive heart failure), such as high BP and cholesterol (because they can aggravate the syndrome), but also to recognise and correct malnutrition and deficiencies in specific micronutrients. Some macronutrients such as essential fatty acids may even be critical.

The main aims of nutritional intervention is the reduction of oedema, the improvement of nutritional status especially in patients with cardiac cachexia and the improvement of respiratory function in patients with dyspnoea. Current congestive heart failure management guidelines indicate that sodium intake levels can range between 2.0 and 2.4 g/day ('restricted') and 3–4 g/day ('moderate restriction'). Foods rich in salt such as cheese, sausages, crisps, tinned soup and vegetables, ham, bacon, tinned meat and tinned or smoked fish should therefore be avoided. Low-sodium bread and other bakery products are preferred. Apart from sodium restriction, a dietitian should also bear in mind other nutrition-related issues for patients with congestive heart failure, such as:

- weight monitoring (both overweight and underweight are common problems)
- fluid retention
- cardiac cachexia
- alcohol restriction
- drug–nutrient interactions
- reduced exercise tolerance
- pre-transplant preparation and post-transplant requirements

Table 6.4 presents the basic nutritional recommendations for congestive heart failure patients. Although there are some studies exploring the effect of

Table 6.4 Dietary recommendations for patients with congestive heart failure.

Nutrient	Recommended intake
Calories	Underweight: 32 kcal/kg body weight
	Normal weight: 28 kcal/kg body weight
Protein	0.8–1 g/kg body weight
	Cardiac cachexia or malnutrition: 1.2–1.5 g/kg body weight
Fat	Saturated <10% of total kcal
	Trans <2% of total kcal
	Omega-3 fatty acids 1.3 g (fish or supplements)
Sodium	2000–2300 mg
	Severe oedema: temporarily 1200–1500 mg
Fluid	Usually 1.5–2 l, depends on oedema and drug therapy

several nutritional supplements (e.g. coenzyme Q10, carnitine, creatine and taurine) in patients with congestive heart failure, the joint American College of Cardiology/American Heart Association guidelines published in 1999 did not support the routine use of such supplements as their safety and efficacy had not been established. To date, there have been no definitive studies to counter their position. Thus, the use of these dietary supplements cannot be recommended at this time.

Further reading

AHA Science Advisory (2001) Stanol/Sterol ester-containing foods and blood cholesterol levels. *Circulation* **103**: 1177–9.

AHA Scientific Statement (2005) Managing abnormal blood lipids. *Circulation* **112**: 3184–209.

AHA Scientific Statement (2006) Diet and lifestyle recommendations revision 2006. *Circulation* **114**: 82–96.

August P (2003) Initial treatment of hypertension. *New England Journal of Medicine* **348**: 610–7.

Beyer FR, Dickinson HO, Nicolson DJ *et al.* (2006) Combined calcium, magnesium and potassium supplementation for the management of primary hypertension in adults. *Cochrane Database of Systematic Reviews 2006*, Issue 3. Art. No.: CD004805. DOI: 10.1002/14651858.CD004805.pub2.

Cornelissen VA, Fagard RH (2005) Effects of endurance training on BP, BP-regulating mechanisms, and cardiovascular risk factors. *Hypertension* **46**(4): 667–75.

Dickinson HO, Mason JM, Nicolson DJ *et al.* (2006) Lifestyle interventions to reduce raised BP: A systematic review of randomized controlled trials. *Journal of Hypertension* **24**(2): 215–33.

Ershow AG, Costello RB (2006) Dietary guidance in heart failure: A perspective on needs for prevention and management. *Heart Failure Reviews* **11**: 7–12.

Expert Panel on Detection, Evaluation, and Treatment of High Blood Cholesterol in Adults (2001) Executive summary of the Third Report of the National Cholesterol Education Program (NCEP) Expert Panel on Detection, Evaluation, and Treatment of High Blood Cholesterol in Adults (Adult Treatment Panel III). *Journal of the American Medical Association* **285**: 2486–97.

von Haehling S, Doehner W, Anker S (2007) Nutrition, metabolism, and the complex pathophysiology of cachexia in chronic heart failure. *Cardiovascular Research* **73**(2): 298–309.

Lennie TA (2006) Nutritional recommendations for patients with heart failure. *Journal of Cardiovascular Nursing* **21**(4): 261–8.

Mancia G, De Backer G, Dominiczak A *et al.* (2007) 2007 Guidelines for the management of arterial hypertension: The Task Force for the Management of Arterial Hypertension of the European Society of Hypertension (ESH) and of the European Society of Cardiology (ESC). *Journal of Hypertension* **28**(12): 1462–536.

National High BP Education Program Working Group report on primary prevention of hypertension (1993) *Archives of Internal Medicine* **153**(2): 186–208.

Neter JE, Stam BE, Kok FJ *et al.* (2003) Influence of weight reduction on BP: A meta-analysis of randomized controlled trials. *Hypertension* **42**(5): 878–84.

Noordzij M, Uiterwaal C, Arends LR (2005) BP response to chronic intake of coffee and caffeine: A meta-analysis of randomized controlled trials. *Journal of Hypertension* **23**(5): 921–8.

Riccardi G, Rivellese AA (2000) Dietary treatment of the metabolic syndrome: The optimal diet. *British Journal of Nutrition* **83**(suppl. 1): S143–8.

Chapter 6

Chapter 7

Gastrointestinal Diseases

Meropi Kontogianni

Upper gastrointestinal system

How can diet restrict symptoms of nausea and vomiting?

In cases of nausea and vomiting, some dietary manipulations, described below, may restrict symptoms; however, patients and therapists should be aware of and closely monitor the patient's hydration status, since dehydration is very common.

Ways of restricting nausea and vomiting

- Avoid drinking fluids with meals. Consume small sips of fluids or with a straw and preferably between meals or 40–60 min before or after them.
- Cold drinks may be better tolerated than warm/hot ones.
- Carbonated drinks or ice cubes may alleviate the sense of nausea.
- Consumption of crackers, low-fat cereal bars, pretzels or toast may restrict nausea, especially during the morning.
- Foods that commonly cause dyspepsia, such as fatty or fried foods, coffee, foods rich in spices or condiments and also vegetables with a strong odour, such as onions, garlic and cruciferous vegetables, should be generally avoided.
- Cold foods and those with a mild odour are better tolerated.
- Small and frequent meals prevent stomach distension, as well as the feeling of emptiness, which often aggravates nausea.
- Avoid smelling food during preparation/cooking.
- Avoid going to bed straight after consuming food.

In the event of repeated vomiting episodes, the consumption of drinks or snacks rich in simple carbohydrates (e.g. sugar, honey, etc.), which are easily digested and quickly absorbed, can provide a significant amount of caloric intake.

Do low-fat diets have a place in gastro-oesophageal reflux disease treatment?

Several physiological studies of human volunteers have shown increased frequency of transient lower oesophageal sphincter relaxation and increased oesophageal acid exposure with high fat consumption. These studies examined both healthy volunteers as well as patients with gastro-oesophageal reflux disease (GERD). However, the reported effects of fatty meals on GERD symptoms remain controversial. Severe fat restriction (i.e. <45 g per day) is not justified, according to scientific data for GERD treatment; however, patients may benefit from a moderate fat diet (~30% of total daily intake), especially those who also suffer from symptoms of dyspepsia and/or delayed gastric emptying.

What lifestyle modifications can alleviate the symptoms of gastro-oesophageal reflux disease?

There are certain modifications to a person's lifestyle that can alleviate the symptoms of GERD, including:

- smoking cessation
- avoidance of excessive coffee intake and other caffeine-containing drinks/foods
- restriction of alcohol and avoidance of alcohol consumption on an empty stomach
- reduced intake of carbonated or acidic juices from citrus fruits
- patients should check whether foods such as citrus fruits, chocolate, fatty and fried foods, garlic and onions, mint flavourings, spicy foods and tomato-based foods (e.g. spaghetti sauce, salsa, chilli) worsen reflux symptoms
- small and frequent meals and avoidance of lying down 2–3 hours after a meal can alleviate symptoms
- if overweight, especially central fat deposition, weight loss may help patients, as will wearing loose-fitting clothes
- sleeping with the upper part of the body raised by 15–20 cm (5.85–7.8 in.) can limit GERD symptoms
- exercise immediately after meal consumption should be avoided.

What are the dietary recommendations during the acute phase of oesophagitis?

In cases of oesophagitis, diet aims at:

- preventing further inflammation of the mucosa

- restricting reflux episodes
- reducing the acidity of gastric juices.

In the acute phase, patients should consume a liquid or soft diet and should avoid acid foods, such as those containing lemon juice, vinegar and soft drinks, spices and condiments (especially red and black pepper, dried red peppers, paprika) as well as alcohol intake. Moreover, all the lifestyle modifications described above for GERD can help patients with oesophagitis.

What are the main nutrition-related problems associated with oesophageal achalasia?

Achalasia is characterised by the failure to relax the lower oesophageal sphincter and the absence of progressive peristalsis in the oesophageal body. Most common symptoms include dysphagia (especially of solid foods), regurgitation, chest pain, heartburn, unintentional weight loss and cough. Aspiration of food from the oesophagus may lead to pneumonia. Sometimes, patients become afraid to eat, and this may result in a deterioration of their nutritional status. Very small and frequent meals are better tolerated, whereas in some cases administration of a liquid diet, rich in energy and protein, is the only solution. Standing up during a meal, drinking a glass of water and exhaling hard may also force food to the stomach. Avoidance of fatty or fried foods that aggravate dyspepsia, restriction of very hot or very cold foods/drinks that increase air ingestion and avoidance of foods or drinks, such as coffee, tea, alcohol, citrus juices or foods with spices that can irritate the mucosa in the event of food stasis in the oesophagus, may offer patients some relief.

What points should dietary advice emphasise after the placement of oesophageal stents?

Dietary advice for these patients should focus on adequate fluids, energy and nutrient intake, as well as on minimising the risk of tube obstruction. During the initiation of the oral diet, the patient should take a clear liquid diet for almost 24 hours. Then a semi-solid soft diet with consumption of small portions of liquids after solid food intake should be prescribed. Patients should avoid hard and dehydrated parts of meat, hard or stringy cheese, breadcrumbs, nuts, raw vegetables, fruit skins, dried fruits and citrus pith and should be very careful with fish bones. Moreover, they should chew small mouthfuls of food thoroughly and drink plenty of fluid. Small and frequent meals are better tolerated, and meals enriched with energy and protein is really important to treat or prevent malnutrition. In cases of continuing dysphagia, the dietitian should modify the diet according to the patient's chewing and swallowing ability and assess their nutritional status on a regular basis.

Chapter 7

Does current scientific evidence support the provision of so-called bland diets in patients with peptic ulcer disease?

In the past, a 'bland diet' was prescribed for patients with peptic ulcer disease. This diet emphasised small and frequent meals, the avoidance of caffeine and spices, a low fibre intake, the avoidance of large quantities of milk and puréed foods in order to avoid any mechanical injury to the stomach. However, recent scientific evidence does not justify the prescription of such a diet, especially since the significant progression of the pharmacological treatment of peptic ulcer disease.

What is the role of dietary management in peptic ulcer disease?

Diet plays a minor role in peptic ulcer treatment and the main aim is to alleviate patients' symptoms, especially at times of exacerbation. There is little clinical evidence about specific foods to avoid and most patients are aware of their intolerances, which may differ significantly among patients with ulcer. Generally, foods that often exacerbate symptoms include spices, especially red hot pepper and paprika, coffee and other caffeine-containing beverages, as well as large amounts of alcoholic beverages. Acid foods, such as vinegar, lemon, orange and other citrus fruits and their juices have been traditionally avoided by patients with peptic ulcer on the grounds that these items exacerbate symptoms. During periods of exacerbation, acid foods should be limited, and patients may benefit from a soft diet, without large amounts of fat or fried foods. The thorough chewing of food, the avoidance of large meals that cause stomach distension and the limited consumption of carbonated drinks may also alleviate symptoms in times of exacerbation; however, patients should be encouraged to consume a balanced diet, including all food groups.

What are the main categories of gastric surgeries?

Nowadays, the most common indicators for gastric surgery are stomach cancer and morbid obesity, whereas surgery for peptic ulcer is seldom due to the effective drug treatment of the disease. The types of surgeries for morbid obesity have been already discussed in Chapter 4. In the case of gastric cancer, the most common surgical procedure is total gastrectomy, although in some cases subtotal gastrectomy is also performed. Moreover, vagotomy or partial Bilroth I and II gastrectomies are the procedures of choice for peptic ulcer disease.

What dietary protocols should patients follow after undergoing gastric surgery?

Right after the surgery, patients should consume nothing orally until the initiation of the intestinal movements. During this period, patients receive fluids and electrolytes parenterally, and in some cases total parenteral nutrition is indicated. When food consumption begins, low-carbohydrate fluids are the first stage (tea, sugar-free jelly, clear fruit juices, vegetables, chicken or beef broth). The next stage, provided that fluids have been well tolerated, involves administering a soft diet, rich in protein [1–1.5 g/kg (0.45–0.68 g/lb) of body weight], low in carbohydrate (especially sugars) and moderate in fat. Small and frequent meals (approximately every two hours) are better tolerated and during the first period of feeding a low-fibre diet and consumption of fluids away from solid food intake benefit patients. Raw fruits and vegetables should be initiated in the diet 2–3 weeks after surgery. Milk and carbonated beverages should be avoided during the short-term post-surgical period in order to avoid gastric distension and dumping syndrome.

What are the principles of dumping syndrome's dietary treatment?

Dumping syndrome describes a combination of symptoms that occur when food is emptied too quickly from the stomach, filling the small intestine with undigested food that is not adequately prepared to permit the efficient absorption of nutrients in the small intestine. Dumping syndrome is most commonly seen after a gastrectomy and its symptoms are divided into early symptoms, which begin during or right after a meal and include nausea, vomiting, bloating, cramping, diarrhoea, dizziness and fatigue, and late symptoms, which occur 1–3 hours after eating and include hypoglycaemia, weakness, sweating and dizziness. People with dumping syndrome often have both types of symptoms. The main dietary guidelines for the prevention and treatment of dumping syndrome include:

- Small and frequent meals (at least six). Slow food consumption and thorough chewing of solid foods. The patient should sit upright while eating and lay down for 30 minutes after meal or snack consumption.
- Fluid consumption during meals should be limited. Liquids should be ingested 30–60 minutes before or after meals instead of with meals. Fluids should be of low osmolarity and not more than 120 ml (4.22 fl oz) each time during the first post-surgical period.
- Foods high in simple sugars should be avoided, because they pass through the stomach quickly and may cause diarrhoea and cramping. Hence, high sugary foods and beverages including fruit juices/drinks, soda, cakes, pies, candy, doughnuts and cookies should be limited or completely avoided.
- Protein should provide about 20% of daily caloric intake for tissue repair and optimal nutritional status. Foods such as milk, yogurt, cottage or other cheese, meat, poultry, fish and egg whites are good protein sources and should be consumed on a daily basis.
- Fat should cover 30–40% of daily caloric intake. Fats slow the stomach emptying and may help to prevent dumping syndrome episodes. Moreover, they are energy dense and may provide a substantial amount of calories for the patient. Butter, margarine, mayonnaise, gravy, vegetable oils, salad dressings and cream cheese are good choices.

Chapter 7

- Fibres should be gradually introduced in the diet. Foods high in soluble fibre (e.g. apples, beets, Brussels sprouts, carrots, oats, spinach, pears) slow stomach emptying and prevent sugars from being absorbed too quickly.
- Milk should be gradually introduced in the diet since some patients develop intolerance. In the event of distress, lactose-free milk may alleviate the symptoms. Patient should, however, ensure the intake of sufficient calcium and vitamin D on a daily basis.
- Fluids and foods should be consumed when they are of a moderate temperature. Cold drinks may substantially increase intestinal motility.
- Avoiding simple sugars and consuming frequent meals provide protection against late dumping syndrome hypoglycaemia; however, in cases of a hypoglycaemic event, the patient should follow the respective instructions as they are described in Chapter 5.

What are the most frequent nutritional deficiencies after gastric surgery?

The main nutrients affected by stomach surgery are protein, vitamin B_{12}, iron and calcium. For this reason, a careful and regular check of these nutrients should be introduced once their deficiencies limit quality of life. Dietitians should emphasise protein intake, especially in cancer patients, whose needs are increased. Provision of a protein supplement or respective guidance for protein fortification of the diet should be administered and nutritional status should be systematically monitored.

Vitamin B_{12} deficiency is common after gastric surgery, mainly when restrictive procedures are involved. The deficiency is due to a failure of separation of vitamin B_{12} from protein foodstuffs and to a failure of absorption of crystalline vitamin B_{12}, since intrinsic factor is not present. Although the body storage of vitamin B_{12} is substantial (about 2000 mg) compared to the smaller, daily needs (2 mg/day), the deficiency is relatively common in patients after 1–9 years of gastric surgery. Close monitoring of vitamin B_{12} levels for the rest of the patient's life is crucial and, in cases of deficiency, the parenteral administration of the vitamin is required. The aetiology of iron deficiency is multifactorial. In order to be absorbed, dietary iron (as ferric ion) must be reduced to the ferrous state by the acid secretion of the stomach. Since there is a reduced production of hydrochloric acid after restrictive procedures, iron is less available to be absorbed. Moreover, in the event of a bypass, with the exclusion of duodenum and proximal jejunum, the main areas of iron's absorption are bypassed. Published recommendations for iron supplementation range from 40 to 65 mg of supplemental iron per day for patients with stomach surgeries.

Finally, patients who have been submitted to restrictive or malabsorptive bariatric surgery are prone to bone mass abnormalities. It is caused by the restriction of calcium intake associated with malabsorption of both calcium and vitamin D. Reduced calcium absorption is secondary to the exclusion of duodenum and proximal jejunum, where calcium is maximally absorbed. Vitamin D is absorbed preferentially in the jejunum and ileum. The defective absorption of fat and fat-soluble vitamins, including vitamin D, aggravates calcium malabsorption. The relative lack of calcium stimulates the production of parathyroid hormone that, in turn, causes the increased production of 1,25-dihydroxyvitamin D and the increased release of calcium from bone. The result of this process is the long-term risk of osteoporosis. Patients should be advised to take 1200–1500 mg of calcium per day and 10 µg of vitamin D.

Lower gastrointestinal system

What should dietary assessment and the counselling of a patient with constipation focus on?

In general, a low-fibre diet, inadequate fluid intake, irregular meals, physical inactivity and/or suppression or ignorance of the urge for defecation are the main lifestyle factors that contribute to constipation and those that dietitians should focus on during the dietary assessment.

During dietary counselling for the prevention and treatment of constipation, patients should be advised to increase fibre intake to at least 25 g per day from fruits, vegetables, wholegrain cereals and legumes. To minimise the risk of flatulence, distension and bloating, fibre intake should be increased gradually over a period of weeks or months. Patients should be encouraged to persist with their new diet as it may take up to a month before they fully benefit from it. Prunes and prune juice contain an ingredient (dihydroxyphenyl isatin) that, according to some scientific evidence, triggers intestinal peristalsis. Moreover, bulking agents such as psyllium hydrophilic mucilloid (ispaghula husk) and wheat bran intake increase faecal volume by absorbing water and so stimulate defecation. The recommended intake for wheat bran varies from one teaspoon to 4–6 tablespoons per day, in parallel with increased fluid intake, and its laxative effect usually appears 12–24 hr after its ingestion. Wheat bran should be avoided in cases of bowel obstruction or atony. Fat addition in the diet may partly alleviate symptoms of constipation owing to cholecystokinin and bile secretion, which in turn increases water absorption in the intestine and hence results in softer stools. Adequate fluid intake and hydration [30–35 ml/kg (0.48–0.56 fl oz/lb) fluid] is very important for normal bowel function, and patients should be aware of this – especially if they increase fibre intake or they are taking fibre supplements.

However, any advice given to patients suffering from constipation must be realistic and tailored to the individual. For example, a fluid intake of two litres per day may be hard to achieve for some older patients or even contraindicated, for example in patients with heart failure. Patients with haemorrhoids should also follow the above-mentioned recommendations in order to avoid constipation and the subsequent swelling and inflammation of blood vessels in the rectum and anus.

What are the main categories of and the nutritional management for diarrhoea?

Diarrhoea is commonly classified in four main categories, namely osmotic (e.g. in carbohydrate malabsorption), secretory (e.g. bacterial infections, microscopic colitis, bile acid malabsorption), inflammatory (e.g. inflammatory bowel disease) and that due to dysmotility (e.g. irritable bowel syndrome). Diarrhoea treatment is based on the treatment of the basic disease which causes the symptom of diarrhoea. The major problem in patients with severe diarrhoea is fluid loss and the concomitant loss of sodium, potassium and bicarbonates, and so their substitution is the first aim in order to prevent dehydration, hyponatraemia, hypokalaemia and acidosis prevention. Fluid repletion is accomplished with fluid administration, either parenterally or orally, rich in electrolytes and carbohydrates. Glucose facilitates the absorption of sodium and other electrolytes and should be included in the hydration solutions.

During the acute phase of diarrhoea, a clear liquid diet should be administered and should be followed by a full liquid and then a soft diet low in fat and fibre, with easily digestible foods (e.g. rice, potatoes, refined cereals). Pectin administration in the form of apple juice or supplement may alleviate the symptoms of diarrhoea. Patients with osmotic diarrhoea should avoid large amounts of fructose, sucrose and lactose. Often, patients with acute diarrhoea develop temporary lactose intolerance owing to partial damage of the intestinal mucosa and a reduction in lactase bioavailability.

In cases of chronic diarrhoea, dietary treatment depends on the underlying cause (e.g. coeliac disease, lactose intolerance, Crohn's disease) and dietitians should emphasise on patient's nutritional status in order to prevent protein-energy malnutrition or micronutrient deficiencies.

Which foods increase gas production in the gastrointestinal tract?

Patients with gastric distension or flatulence may alleviate their symptoms by reducing the intake of the following foods that produce gas in the gastrointestinal tract:

- beans, peas, lentils
- cabbage, cauliflower, broccoli, onions, turnips, cucumber, okra, corn
- prunes, apples, raisins
- wheat bran, excessive quantities of wheat products or fruits
- sugar substitutes (e.g. sorbitol, manitol) when consumed in large quantities.
- lactose-rich foods

What are the properties and use of medium-chain triglycerides?

Medium-chain triglycerides (MCTs) are triglycerides with 8–12 carbons per molecule that do not form micelles in order to be digested and therefore do not need the presence of bile acids for their metabolism and absorption. MCTs give 8.3 kcal/g (34.75 kJ/g), are absorbed in the small intestine and are delivered in the liver through the portal vein, where they are further metabolised. MCTs are usually administered in cases of reduced fat absorption (e.g. steatorrhoea, AIDS, short bowel syndrome, severe acute pancreatitis, hyperchylomicronaemia, bile acid deficiency) in order to provide patients with extra calories. MCTs are usually available in the form of oil that can be used in salads, dressings, sausages and juices, but not for cooking in high temperatures, such as frying and cannot be used as the only source of fat since they do not contain essential fatty acids and fat-soluble vitamins. The use of MCTs may also exhibit some side effects, namely gastric cramps, nausea and diarrhoea, if they are consumed in high quantities. Hence, MCTs should be gradually introduced into the diet and be evenly distributed throughout the day, avoiding more than 15 g of MCTs per meal.

How can patients with lactose intolerance fulfil their calcium needs?

Patients with lactose intolerance cannot digest milk and sometimes yoghurt; however, most patients can tolerate cheese, especially hard cheese, which contains very small quantities of lactose and is usually very rich in calcium (e.g. parmesan, cheddar). In order to fulfil their calcium needs, patients can also try lactose-free milk, cruciferous vegetables (e.g. cauliflower, cabbage, Brussels sprouts), tinned fish containing soft bones such as salmon, small fishes that contain small bones such as whitebait and sprats, mineral water rich in calcium, fortified industry products or calcium supplements.

What is coeliac disease and how is it treated?

Coeliac disease results from the interaction between gluten and immune, genetic and environmental factors and is precipitated by the ingestion of gluten, the major storage protein of wheat and similar grains, which is derived from wheat, barley and rye. The gluten protein is rich in glutamine and proline and is poorly digested in the upper gastrointestinal tract. These peptides pass through the epithelial barrier of the intestine, possibly during intestinal infections or when there is an increase in intestinal permeability, and interact with antigen-presenting cells in the lamina propria. Coeliac disease is characterised by diarrhoea, emaciation, aphthous stomatitis and malabsorption. However, vomiting, irritability, anorexia and even constipation are also common. Older children, adolescents and adults often present disease with extraintestinal manifestations only, such as short stature, neurological symptoms or anaemia.

Nutritional therapy is the only accepted treatment for coeliac disease and involves the lifelong elimination of wheat, rye and barley from the diet. Clinical studies suggest that oats are tolerated by most patients with coeliac disease and may improve the nutritional content of their diet and overall quality of life. However, oats are not uniformly recommended, because most

Chapter 7

commercially available oats are contaminated with gluten-containing grains during the growing, transportation and milling processes. Although wheat, rye and barley should be completely avoided, there are other foods and grains, such as rice, corn and potato, that can serve as substitutes as well as other sources of starch that can provide flours for cooking and baking. Because the substitute flours are not fortified with B vitamins, vitamin deficiencies may occur and they have been detected in patients who are on the diet for a long time (more than 10 years). Therefore, vitamin supplementation is advised. Meats, dairy products, fruit and vegetables are naturally gluten-free and help to make for a more nutritious and varied diet, and there is a great variety of specially manufactured gluten-free products that are usually prescribed to coeliac patients. Table 7.1 describes the most common sources of gluten as well as gluten-free foods. Problems often arise from 'hidden gluten', since many commercial products, ready meals, convenience foods and occasionally some medications have wheat flour or other gluten-containing starches added as filler, thickener or stabilising agents.

After a diagnosis of coeliac disease has been established, the patient should be assessed for deficiencies of vitamins and minerals, including folic acid, B_{12}, fat-soluble vitamins, iron and calcium, and any deficiency observed should be treated. All patients with coeliac disease should undergo screening for osteoporosis, which has a high prevalence in this population. Lifelong adherence to the diet even in latent or silent forms of the disease is crucial since it significantly reduces patients' morbidity and mortality, and dietitians should strive for patient compliance to the diet.

What are the main reasons for malnutrition in patients with inflammatory bowel disease?

Several mechanisms contribute to the malnutrition observed in inflammatory bowel disease (IBD) patients. A decrease in the oral intake of nutrients is a common symptom and is often due to abdominal pain, diarrhoea, anorexia, nausea and vomiting and in cases of strictures or abscesses. Moreover, mucosal inflammation and its associated diarrhoea or bleeding lead to a loss of protein, blood, minerals, electrolytes and trace elements. Multiple resections, bacterial overgrowth and fistulas between the small and large intestine may have an adverse nutritional effect (e.g. vitamins and minerals) owing to a decreased absorptive area and subsequent malabsorption. Furthermore, increased energy requirements because of inflammation or fever can lead to weight loss and altered intermediate metabolism, owing to increased TNF-alpha, IL-1 and 6, which in turn lead to decreased albumin and other protein synthesis. Pharmacological therapies may also lead to malnutrition. For example, sulfasalazine reduces folic acid absorption, whereas corticosteroids decrease calcium absorption and negatively affect protein metabolism. Lastly, restrictive diets that are recommended to patients by family, friends and physicians or prolonged periods of fasting because of exacerbations or diagnostic procedures also contribute to the risk of malnutrition. The

Table 7.1 Common sources of gluten in foods.

Gluten-free foods	Foods containing gluten
Cereals and flour Rice, rice flour, rice bran, corn (maize), cornflour, cornmeal, arrowroot, buckwheat, millet, quinoa, sorghum, soya flour, potato starch, potato flour, gram flour (chick pea), polenta, sago, tapioca and cassava.	Wheat, barley, rye, oats and their flours, Kamut, bulgar wheat, durum wheat, couscous, wheat bran, wheat germ.
Breakfast cereals Rice-based breakfast cereals, corn-based breakfast cereals, buckwheat flakes.	All wheat-based breakfast cereals. Muesli.
Breads, cakes and biscuits Specially manufactured gluten-free breads, biscuits, cakes, pizza bases, rolls, flour mixes, rice cakes, meringues and macaroons.	All ordinary bread and bread products, croissants, bagels, brioche, pitta bread. Ordinary cakes, biscuits, crackers, pastries & crumbles, pizza, croutons, and batter.
Pasta Corn pasta, rice pasta, rice noodles, specially manufactured gluten-free pasta.	All fresh, dried and canned pasta. Noodles.
Meat and poultry All fresh meat and poultry prepared without gravy or sauce, meat canned or pre-packed in its own juices or jelly, bacon, sausages that are 100% meat.	Meat pies, sausages, meat and poultry prepared with gravy or sauce or breadcrumbs.
Fish Fish prepared without sauces, batter or breadcrumbs, fish canned in oil or brine.	Fish fingers, fish in batter or breadcrumbs, fish cakes.
Dairy products and eggs Milk, yoghurt, fromage frais, cheese, goat's and sheep's milk, soya milk, buttermilk, margarine, oil, butter, low-fat spreads, milk puddings (rice, cream), eggs.	Yoghurts containing muesli or cereal, cheese spread and processed cheese, Scotch eggs.
Vegetables and fruits All fruits and vegetables, potatoes including oven chips, microwave and frozen chips.	Potato croquettes, chips coated with added flour.
Miscellaneous Sugar, jams, marmalade, jelly, sorbets. Salt, pepper, herbs, spices. Tea, coffee, fruit juices, fruit squash, clear fizzy drinks, cocoa. Wine, spirits, cider, sherry, port, liqueurs.	Stuffing, soy sauce. Malted milk drinks. Barley water and cloudy fizzy drinks. Beer, lager, stout, real ale.

Chapter 7

consequences of malnutrition are numerous, and include reductions in bone mineral density, as well as growth retardation and delayed sexual maturity in children. Osteoporosis may also be implicated as a result of pro-inflammatory cytokine profiles.

What are the main nutritional deficiencies of inflammatory bowel disease?

IBD is associated with a number of nutritional deficiencies, including anaemia, hypoalbuminaemia, hypomagnesaemia, hypocalcaemia and hypophosphataemia, as well as deficiencies in folic acid, niacin, fat-soluble vitamins and B_{12} in cases of terminal ileum resection and deficiencies of iron, zinc and copper. Plasma antioxidant concentrations are also reduced in many IBD patients, particularly those with active disease. Patients with diarrhoea and vomiting may also experience electrolyte imbalances.

What kind of diet should be administered to a patient with ulcerative colitis exacerbation?

For nutritional support, enteral feeds are generally preferred to parenteral nutrition, except from cases of toxic megacolon, extended colon haemorrhage, perforation or obstruction, which require bowel rest and parenteral administration of fluids and nutrients. In times of exacerbation, a liquid diet is first administered, followed by a low-residue diet. In patients with strictures, a low-fibre diet is required in order to prevent obstruction. When the patient enters the remission phase, they should be encouraged to consume a variety of foods from all food groups and dietitians should help patients realise their own intolerances and further compose a balanced diet.

Which are the main dietary goals in the management of Crohn's disease?

Medical nutritional therapy for patients with Crohn's disease (CD) aims to:

- prevent or restore protein/energy malnutrition
- assess and correct micronutrient deficiencies
- maintain bowel rest in periods of exacerbation
- modify the diet regime according to drug treatment and drug–nutrient interactions
- modulate immune response by modulating cytokines expression (e.g. omega-3 polyunsaturated fatty acids), by reducing gut permeability and enhancing gut barrier (e.g. probiotics), by affecting gene expression (e.g. polyunsaturated fatty acids have dramatic effects on gene expression through the regulation of several transcription factors, including peroxisome proliferator-activated receptors, or PPAR) and by modulating local immunity in the intestine (e.g. butyrate, glutamine).

What are the protein and energy requirements in Crohn's disease during the exacerbation phase?

Adults with no signs of malnutrition will need 25–30 kcal/kg (47.6–57.1 kJ/lb) body weight, whereas individuals with malnutrition may need 30–35 kcal/kg body weight. Protein requirements range from 1 to 1.5 g/kg (0.45–0.68 g/lb) body weight, but may reach 2 g/kg (0.91 g/lb), especially in malnutrition or septic conditions. Adequate fluid intake is also crucial because of increased fluid loss. Patients should receive about 35 ml/kg (0.56 fl oz/lb) body weight plus the estimated losses from diarrhoea, fever, fistulas, etc.

When is total parenteral nutrition indicated in inflammatory bowel disease patients?

Total parenteral nutrition (TPN) has a role in patients with a non-functioning intestine or with short bowel syndrome due to excessive resections. Additionally, TPN aims at preoperative bowel rest, fulfilling postoperative nutritional requirements and correcting malnutrition. TPN can also be used as a primary therapy for active and severe IBD, since bowel rest is believed to improve the control of intestinal inflammation by reducing the presence of antigens and bacterial growth in the lumen, by reducing peristaltic movements and digestive tract secretion and by leading to the relief of symptoms. In other cases, TPN can be used as a complement to poorly tolerated or quantitatively insufficient oral or enteral nutrition to maintain the patient's nutritional status or to correct malnutrition. Malnutrition-related complications occur in a significant number of IBD patients after surgical treatment. Reduction of these complications with at least five days of preoperative TPN is well observed in patients with severe malnutrition, presenting with low serum albumin (<3.5 g/dl) and transferrin (<150 mg/dl) levels. In these situations, TPN provides nutritional requirements, preserves lean body mass and functional capacity and prevents protein loss in acute disease course. Furthermore, fistulas due to CD are common, because of transmural inflammation, and numerous reports about the effects of TPN in intestinal fistulas reveal initial closure rates of up to 44%. TPN is also indicated in cases of intestinal obstruction and in perianal CD, for which treatment is usually conservative owing to frequent recurrences and the possible involvement of sphincter muscles. Nonetheless, TPN adds significant cost and length to hospital admissions, especially when septic, metabolic or venous access complications occur, and the scientific data so far indicate that TPN should be offered to IBD patients in need of nutritional therapy who do not tolerate the enteral route, especially during acute and severe disease courses.

When is enteral nutrition indicated in patients with inflammatory bowel disease and what type of formula is preferred?

In IBD, enteral nutrition (EN) is provided in general to correct nutritional deficits or to serve as primary therapy for clinically active disease. Total EN

Chapter 7

excludes potential toxic dietary factors and antigenic exposure, since it consists of amino acids, glucose or oligosaccharides and has a low lipid content. When compared to TPN, EN yielded similar results for the prevention and combating of malnutrition. EN is easier to use, is less expensive and is a better alternative to TPN. Unfortunately, its unpalatability limits patient compliance, but with strong encouragement this may be partially overcome. Regarding enteral nutrition type, polymeric diets are most often prescribed, mainly in patients with adequate gastrointestinal function. Elemental diets contain nutrients in their simple form, being historically indicated for patients with malabsorption. Intolerance to polymeric diets and short bowel syndrome are the main indications to semi-elemental and elemental formulas. Elemental diets were also introduced as primary treatment for active CD because of their low allergenic capacity, providing lower antigenic (since they don't have integral proteins or peptides) and inflammatory stimulation. As absorbed by the proximal jejunum, elemental diets provide nutrients and trophic stimuli for this segment, keeping the distal small bowel and colon (the most common sites of CD activity) at relative rest. Elemental and semi-elemental diets also reduce the bacterial load and hence decrease intestinal permeability. Elemental and polymeric diets can, in many cases, induce active CD remission; however, there aren't enough data to support the substitution of drug therapy by EN.

In conclusion, recent literature reviews and meta-analyses of controlled randomised trials have not shown any significant difference between elemental, oligomeric and polymeric diets concerning initial or late remission of active CD, even though elemental diets are related to earlier remission. Polymeric diets should be preferentially used in the treatment of acute CD, as they offer lower costs, better patient tolerance and the possibility of immunological action of their contents. In general, EN should be preferred to TPN in nutritional therapy. As primary therapy to active CD, data suggest that EN's efficacy is equal to that of TPN, but it is less effective compared to corticosteroids. EN plays an important role in selected cases unresponsive to usual treatment and in children/teenagers, since it is associated with greater linear growth.

Would patients with inflammatory bowel disease benefit from supplements of omega-3 fatty acids or pro/prebiotics?

It has been proposed that supplemental omega-3 fatty acids may be beneficial in treating or preventing relapse in chronic inflammatory diseases. Studies that have examined fatty acid profiles in IBD patients have shown decreased total serum polyunsaturated fatty acids, as well as deficiencies, specifically in omega-3 fatty acids in CD patients. Moreover, evidence exists that a proportion of IBD patients have essential fatty acid deficiency, which can contribute to the pathology of IBD. At the cellular level, IBD is characterised by elevated concentrations of IL-1 and pro-inflammatory leukotriene B (synthesised from omega-6 fatty acids). Immunomodulatory mechanisms proposed for omega-3 fatty acids in IBD include altering eicosanoid synthesis, cell membrane fluidity, cell signal transduction, intraluminal bacterial content and gene expression. Several clinical trials have been conducted to test the effects of omega-3 fatty acid supplements on clinical outcomes, namely clinical scores, endoscopic scores, histological scores, relapse, remission and corticosteroid requirements in IBD. The available data are insufficient to draw conclusions about the effects of omega-3 fatty acids on clinical, endoscopic and histological scores or induced remission and relapse rates. However, the data that pertain to the effects of omega-3 fatty acids on steroid requirements suggest that omega-3 fatty acids may reduce the need for or effective dose of corticosteroids among patients with IBD. Enteric-coated omega-3 fatty acids seem to be more efficient; however, further well-designed studies are needed to assess omega-3 efficacy in IBD treatment.

Moreover, clinical observations suggest that certain intestinal and extraintestinal bacterial infections sometimes precede or reactivate chronic intestinal inflammation. A number of microbial agents may be implicated as initiating factors in the pathogenesis of IBD. Although it is unclear whether the abnormal composition of the enteric flora contribute to the pathogenesis of IBD, evidence from animal models and clinical observations (e.g. antibiotics are effective in certain patients) have prompted the examination of a wide variety of probiotic strains (e.g. *Lactobacillus GG, E. coli strain Nissle 1917, Saccharomyces boulardii, VSL#3*, a mixture of four lactobacilli strains) in the treatment of IBD. Although the results of clinical trials are promising, the current consensus is that a number of larger controlled trials are necessary before the use of probiotics as a routine medical treatment is warranted. Finally, prebiotics are food ingredients not digested or absorbed in the upper intestinal tract that are fermented by intestinal bacteria in a selective way, promoting changes in the gut's ecosystem. Experimental and human studies have shown that inulin and oligofructose stimulate saccharolysis in the colonic lumen and favour the growth of indigenous lactobacilli and bifidobacteria. These effects are associated with reduced mucosal inflammation in animal models of IBD. Strong experimental evidence supports the hypothesis that inulin and oligofructose can offer an opportunity to prevent or mitigate intestinal inflammatory lesions in human CD, ulcerative colitis and pouchitis. Encouraging results have been obtained in preliminary clinical trials, but further studies are necessary.

Chapter 7

What nutritional care for diverticulosis and diverticulitis should be given?

Diverticular disease is one of the most prevalent medical conditions that affect Western populations. Symptomatic diverticular disease can range from mild, low-level symptomatology similar to that seen in irritable bowel syndrome (including pain, flatulence, gastric distension, alternating episodes of constipation or diarrhoea) to acute bouts of diverticulitis, complicated by abscess or frank perforation.

For patients with diverticulosis, diet aims to treat the symptoms, whereas a general recommendation is the increase in fibre intake up to 25–30 g per day, in parallel with an increased fluid intake, in order to increase faeces volume and to reduce intra-intestinal pressure and therefore limit the development of new diverticulae. Furthermore, high-fat meals may induce gut muscle contractions and a feeling of discomfort in patients with diverticular disease and fat reduction in the diet may alleviate symptoms in some patients.

In the case of diverticulitis, initial management includes antibiotics and bowel rest. During the first days, the patient will receive fluids and electrolytes parenterally. When oral feeds begin, a clear liquid diet should be administered. Usually, the patient's symptoms improve within 48–72 hours after admission, after which a low-residue diet can be administered with a gradual increase in fibre intake. Avoidance of nuts, popcorn and sunflower, pumpkin, caraway and sesame seeds has been recommended by physicians out of fear that food particles could enter, block or irritate the diverticula. However, no scientific data support this treatment measure. The seeds in tomatoes, zucchini, cucumbers, strawberries and raspberries, as well as poppy seeds, are generally considered harmless.

What are the clinical symptoms of irritable bowel syndrome?

Irritable bowel syndrome (IBS) is a clinical diagnosis based on symptoms in the absence of organic disease. The cause of IBS is not yet known. Suggestions include psychosocial factors, altered gastrointestinal motility, a heightened sensory function of the intestine or malfermentation of food residues. Typical symptoms include abdominal pain, excessive flatus and variable bowel habit (constipation, diarrhoea or alternation between these two conditions) for which no endoscopic, radiological, histological, biochemical or microbiological cause is apparent.

Which dietary recommendations would alleviate symptoms of irritable bowel syndrome?

Approximately 60% of IBS patients believe that food exacerbates their symptoms, and research has suggested that allergies to certain foods could trigger IBS symptoms. Studies have reported a positive response to elimination diets in 12.5–67% of patients, but the absence of control groups makes it unclear whether these rates simply reflect a placebo response. Moreover, there is no correlation between foods that patients identify as a cause of their IBS symptoms and the results of food allergy testing. An elimination diet avoiding suspected foods or a modified exclusion diet followed by a stepwise re-introduction of foods as described by Parker and colleagues may be useful, but may be too time-consuming for most clinical practice and will be subject to the difficulties of interpretation. Eliminating one food or food group at a time may uncover a food intolerance that is helpful to some IBS patients. However, it will probably not help those who react adversely to more than one food and should be done with the guidance of a registered dietitian. Care should be taken that the patient is maintaining a nutritionally adequate intake and does not have or develop an eating disorder. A careful history is essential and, for many patients, a diary of foods eaten and symptoms experienced will be helpful. Taking note of foods that seem to be followed by increased symptoms within 1–3 days and paying particular attention to milk, lactose, fructose, sorbitol, gas-forming foods (e.g. beans, Brussels sprouts, onions, celery, carrots, raisins, bananas, prune juice, apricots, wheat germ and bagels), wheat, fat and coffee may be useful. In January 2009 an American College of Gastroenterology (ACG) task force updated an evidence-based position statement on the management of irritable bowel syndrome, according to which: 'Patients often believe that certain foods exacerbate their IBS symptoms. There is, however, insufficient evidence that food allergy testing or exclusion diets are efficacious in IBS and their routine use outside of a clinical trial is not recommended (Grade 2C).'

With regard to dietary fibre supplements studied in patients with IBS, these include mostly wheat and corn bran (rich in insoluble fibre), whereas bulking agents include psyllium hydrophilic mucilloid (ispaghula husk), partially hydrolysed guar gum, fructo-oligosaccharide, oligosaccharide, and calcium polycarbophil, all rich in soluble fibres. For some patients with IBS, especially those with constipation, improvement can be achieved by increasing the intake of soluble fibre by 10 to 20 g/day in the form of supplements such as ispaghula, psyllium and probably other supplements and foods high in soluble fibre. Increasing the amount of insoluble fibre in the diet, especially in patients without constipation, may worsen IBS symptoms. According to the previously mentioned position statement: 'Psyllium hydrophilic mucilloid (ispaghula husk) is moderately effective and can be given a conditional recommendation (Grade 2C). A single study reported improvement with calcium polycarbophil. Wheat bran or corn bran is no more effective than placebo in the relief of global symptoms of IBS and cannot be recommended for routine use (Grade 2C).'

Probiotics possess a number of properties that may prove of benefit to patients with IBS. Interpretation of the available literature on the use of probiotics in IBS, however, is hampered by difficulties in comparing studies using probiotics that varied widely in terms of species, strains, preparations and doses. The usefulness of probiotics in the form of foods such as live-culture yogurt, buttermilk, sour poi or miso for IBS symptoms is unproven. Moreover, 'in single organism studies, lactobacilli do not appear effective for patients with IBS; bifidobacteria and certain combinations of probiotics demonstrate some efficacy (Grade 2C),' according to the ACG task force.

Table 7.2 summarises the most common and reliable dietary interventions for patients with IBS.

What is short bowel syndrome?

Short bowel syndrome (SBS) is a complex entity that is due to anatomical or functional loss of part of the small bowel. Patients will present with severe metabolic and nutritional impairments due to a reduction of the effective absorptive surface area of the gut. SBS is one of the causes of a larger entity known as 'intestinal failure' and is a chronic malabsorptive state. Currently, mesenteric vascular accidents are the main cause of SBS in adults, followed by IBD and radiation enteritis, whereas in children, the main causes are congenital and perinatal diseases. The clinical picture associated with SBS varies

Chapter 7

Table 7.2 Common dietary interventions in irritable bowel syndrome, according to patients' symptoms.

Symptoms	Dietary advice
Constipation	High fibre diet (~25 g/day or 14 g/1000 kcal) Increase fluid intake (35 ml/kg body weight) If associated with gas/bloating emphasise soluble fibre and decrease insoluble fibre
	Consider soluble fibre supplement Daily use of peppermint oil may relieve symptoms
Diarrhoea	Exclude food intolerance (e.g. lactose, gluten) Reduce dietary fibre, especially insoluble and resistant starches
	Assess intake of common gastrointestinal irritants (e.g. insoluble fibre, coffee, spicy food, alcohol, sorbitol/fructose)
Flatulence/distension	Exclude lactose intolerance Restrict gas-producing foods (e.g. beans, Brussels sprouts, onions, celery, wheat germ)
	Assess fructose and fructo-oligosaccharides intake Reduce insoluble fibres and resistant starch Daily use of peppermint oil may relieve symptoms

according to the length and location of the affected small bowel, the presence of underlying disease, the presence or absence of the large bowel and ileocecal valve, and the nature of the underlying disease. A combination of diarrhoea, nutrient malabsorption, dysmotility and bowel dilatation may constitute the clinical symptomatology of this syndrome. The remaining bowel undergoes a process called 'adaptation' by which, for 1–2 years, intestinal absorption is re-established to a situation similar to that prior to intestinal resection and is a key factor in determining whether a patient with SBS will progress to intestinal failure and depend on lifelong total parenteral nutrition. Chronic complications of the syndrome include nutrient, electrolyte and vitamin deficiencies.

What factors affect the severity of short bowel syndrome?

The most important factors affecting the severity of SBS and the type of nutritional support necessary to treat it are:

- the length of the remaining small intestine
- the part of the small intestine that has been removed
- functionality and adaptation of the remaining intestine
- maintenance or removal of the large intestine
- maintenance or not of the ileocecal valve
- presence of ileostomy/colostomy or anastomosis
- patient's age.

What route of nutritional support is preferred for patients with short bowel syndrome during the first postoperative period and what are the patient's energy and protein needs?

Patients with SBS will generally require parenteral nutrition for the first 7–10 days following massive enterectomy, whereas for some parenteral nutrition from a central vein may last up to three months, postoperatively. Nutritional therapy, even parenteral nutrition, should be initiated when the patient is haemodynamically stable and fluid management issues are relatively stable. SBS patients would be expected to differ in their response to dietary manipulation depending upon their bowel's anatomy, specifically, the presence or absence of a colon. Patients with less than 100 cm of small intestine around the Treitz ligament and without a large bowel will need parenteral nutrition for an unknown period. Conversely, 50 cm (19.5 in.) of small intestine can be enough for oral feeding after a period of bowel adaptation provided that the ileocecal valve is intact, as well as a big part of the large intestine. The large intestine is a very important organ since after the adaptation phase it can absorb significant amounts of proteins, fluids and electrolytes. Moreover, it can save significant amounts of energy through the conversion of complex carbohydrates to short-chain fatty acids under the activity of the gut flora. The gradual initiation of standard enteral formulas is the next step and once the patient is able to eat they should be encouraged to do so. During the acute post-surgical phase, individual calorie goals can generally be estimated using the calculated resting energy expenditure (e.g. Harris-Benedict or Schofield equations) multiplied by activity and malabsorption factors or by providing 25–35 kcal/kg (47.6–66.6 kJ/lb) body weight [with a mean of 32 kcal/kg (60.9 kJ/lb)]. Protein requirements range from 1 to 1.5 g/kg (0.45–0.68 g/lb) body weight, since nitrogen absorption is least affected by the decreased absorptive surface in SBS patients, and for this reason the use of peptide-based diets in these patients is unnecessary.

What are the major nutritional issues during the late postoperative phase for patients with short bowel syndrome?

In general, most stable adult SBS patients absorb only about one-half to two-thirds as much energy as normal; thus, dietary intake must be increased by at least 50% (i.e. hyperphagic diet). The increased quantity of food tends to be best tolerated when consumed throughout the day in five or six meals. Supplemental tube feeding may be useful in selected patients of any age to meet their caloric needs, particularly when trying to wean parenteral nutrition. Clinical experience suggests that nocturnal gastric tube feeding of a semi-elemental or polymeric formula administered continuously via an infusion pump in small quantities may be better tolerated than bolus tube feeding owing to the greater absorption of nutrients and a reduced occurrence of osmotic diarrhoea. Table 7.3 refers to basic nutritional tips for the dietary management of SBS patients and Table 7.4 describes the recommended nutritional intake when oral nutrition is introduced.

Chapter 7

Table 7.3 Basic nutritional tips for the dietary management of short bowel syndrome patients.

Restricted ileum resection with or without colectomy
Patients with remaining small intestine of 100–150 cm will need total parenteral nutrition for a short period, especially if postsurgical complications are present. Patients with a remaining small intestine of 150–200 cm usually cover their needs with oral feeding and the consumption of oral supplements.
1st step: Initiation of enteral nutrition during the late postsurgery phase.
2nd step: Start per os liquids up to 500 ml/day.
3d step: Progress to small meals of solid food (generally low in fat and fibre, sometimes also low in lactose).

General comments
● Avoid caffeine-containing beverages and foods.
● In the case of steatorrhoea, restrict fat intake, introduce medium-chain triglycerides.
● Gradually introduce soluble fibres.
● Systematic monitoring of vitamin B_{12} concentration.

Extensive small bowel resection and partial colectomy
To initiate enteral nutrition at least 50 cm of jejunum in continuation with large intestine, or in the case of full colectomy at least 100 cm of jejunum, are necessary.
1st step: Start clear liquid diet in parallel with parenteral nutrition (up to 500 ml/day in the first days).
2nd step: Progress to low-fat, high-carbohydrate diet.

General comments
● Malabsorption of bile acids and vitamin $B_{12.}$
● In the case of steatorrhoea, malabsorption of fat-soluble vitamins (A, D, E, K), calcium and magnesium.
● Increased risk for bacterial overgrowth when ileocecal valve is lost.

Extensive small bowel resection and complete colectomy
In this case, the duodenum and a small part of the jejunum are only present.

● When less than 100 cm of functional jejunum is present, the patient will need lifelong total parenteral nutrition. In these patients, even small amounts of food can provoke massive bowel secretions and large stoma outputs, creating a significant risk of hydration. Nutritional deficiencies and electrolyte imbalances are very common.
● For patients with jejunum more than 100 cm:
   ○ Energy needs: 30–60 kcal/kg body weight
   ○ Protein needs: 1.2–1.5 g/kg body weight
   ○ When enteral nutrition is initiated: choose a feed providing 1 kcal/ml or with 300 mOsm/l osmolality. Avoid elemental formulas.
   ○ In patients with an end jejunostomy, avoid enteric formula with fibres.
   ○ Avoid medium-chain triglycerides because they often increase stoma output.
   ○ Avoid caffeine, and large doses of sorbitol, xylitol, mannitol and maybe lactose, owing to their laxative effect.

Table 7.4 Recommended nutrient intake for patients with short bowel syndrome.

Nutrient	Colon present	Colon absent
Protein	20–30% of daily caloric intake	20–30% of daily caloric intake
Carbohydrate	50–60% of daily caloric intake	40–50% of daily caloric intake
	Emphasis on complex CHO	Emphasis on complex CHO
Fat	20–30% of daily caloric intake	30–40% of daily caloric intake
	MCT and LCT	LCT
	Ensure essential fatty acids intake	Ensure essential fatty acids intake
Fibre	Soluble	Soluble
Fluids	30–35 ml/kg body weight	30–35 ml/kg body weight (+ losses)
	Oral rehydration solution	
	Avoid hyperosmolar fluids	Oral rehydration solution
		Avoid hyperosmolar fluids
Oxalates	Restrict	No restriction

CHO: carbohydrate; MCT: medium-chain triglycerides; LCT: long-chain triglycerides.

The optimal fluid components of the diet also depend upon the remaining bowel anatomy. SBS patients without a colon generally require the use of a glucose-electrolyte oral rehydration solution to enhance absorption and reduce secretion, whereas most patients with a colon can maintain adequate hydration with hypotonic fluids. Regardless of bowel anatomy, hyperosmolar fluids such as regular soda and fruit juices should be avoided, as they will aggravate stool losses. Clinical experience suggests that those patients who tend to experience bowel movements shortly after eating (i.e. dumping syndrome) may benefit from avoiding drinking fluids during meals. Parenteral fluids will be necessary if the ostomy output continues to exceed fluid intake.

Moreover, complex carbohydrates reduce the osmotic load and potentially exert a positive effect on the adaptation process. Because the proximal jejunum is rarely resected in SBS patients, lactose is generally well tolerated and should not be restricted unless the patient is clearly intolerant. Concentrated sugars, and fruit juices in particular, should be avoided as they generate a high osmotic load and potentiate stool output. Supplements of soluble fibres may be useful given their potential effect of enhancing adaptation and slowing gastric emptying; however, they may promote increased gas and bloating in the patient.

What dietary modifications are needed in the short term after large bowel resection?

During the first days, parenteral nutrition should be administered in order to cover post-surgical patients' needs both in nutrients and in fluids/electrolytes. Once intestinal movements begin, a clear liquid diet can be introduced, and if patients react normally to the ingestion of liquids, a low-residue and then a low-fibre diet should be administered. Emphasis should be placed on fluid intake in order to ensure adequate hydration and optimum bowel function.

Chapter 7

What are the main nutritional care issues for a patient with an ostomy?

In the case of ileostomy, large bowel resection entails a reduction in water and electrolyte absorption, especially sodium. During the first 6–8 weeks, the stoma output ranges from 1200 to 2000 ml/day (42.23–70.39 fl oz/day) and then is usually reduced as the ileum adapts to the new conditions. At this time, a normal stoma output ranges from 500 to 600 ml/day (17.6–21.11 fl oz/day). If it exceeds 1000–1200 ml/day (35.19–42.23 fl oz/day), the ingestion of isotonic fluids should be increased, as well as the intake of sodium and sugars. Furthermore, the increased intake of fluids and sodium is necessary when the environmental temperature is high, as well as in the case of vomiting or diarrhoea, when increased potassium intake (through the ingestion of fruit juices) and sodium intake (mainly through an increase in added salt) are recommended. Patients with ileostomy who have also undergone terminal ileum resection may need supplemental administration of vitamin B_{12}.

In patients with colostomy, fluids and electrolyte losses depend on the part of the intestine that the stoma has been placed and the major losses are observed when colostomy is placed in the ascending colon.

During the postoperative period, patients with either ileostomy or colostomy will start oral feeding with a clear and then full liquid diet and afterwards feeding progresses to a low-fibre diet ($\leq$10 g of fibre/day). The diet is gradually enriched and the patient will finally follow a normal diet without dietary restrictions. The only problem that can emerge is the stoma obstruction due to undigested parts of food, and in this case a low-residue diet should be administered until the obstruction is resolved. Box 7.1 refers to common dietary advice for patients with an ostomy.

Box 7.1 Basic dietary advice for patients with an ostomy.

- Gradual food re-introduction and progression from a liquid to a normal diet.
- Thorough chewing of foods such as mushrooms, corn, legumes and peppers to prevent stoma obstruction.
- Avoidance of foods such as nuts, tomato skin, pomegranates, figs, okras and the pith of oranges and grapefruits that can block stoma.
- Increase in fluid intake.
- Restriction of foods that can cause unpleasant odours, such as onion, garlic, legumes, egg, fish and cruciferous vegetables.
- In case a patient complains of constipation, diarrhoea or distension/flatulence the respective recommendations should be administered.

Hepatobiliary diseases and exocrine pancreas

What are the main hepatic functions?

The liver is an organ with multiple functions, the most important of which can be summarised as follows:

- the secretion and excretion of substances
- immunomodulatory function (Kupffer cells)
- blood storage
- control of active (toxic) substances through the glutathione antioxidant system or other enzymes
- oxidation and/or reduction of substances, formation of active or inactive metabolites
- concerning nutrients:
  - ○ synthesises bile salts from cholesterol and secretes them in bile. The liver also extracts reabsorbed bile salts from the portal vein blood and returns them to the biliary tree. Hepatic synthesis of bile salts replenishes the fraction of the bile salt pool that escapes re-absorption and is excreted in the faeces.
  - ○ constitutes a major site of fatty acid breakdown and triglyceride synthesis. It stores fat, synthesises cholesterol, performs ketogenesis and forms lipoproteins.
  - ○ regulates the synthesis, storage and breakdown of glycogen (glycogenesis, glycogenolysis), a polymeric form of glucose and also possess enzymes that enable hepatocytes to synthesise glucose from various precursors such as amino acids, pyruvate and lactate (gluconeogenesis).
  - ○ plays central role in the synthesis and degradation of protein. Plasma proteins, including albumin, coagulation factors, transferrin and ceruloplasmin, constitute about one-half of the protein synthesised in the liver. Protein synthesis in the liver is influenced by nutritional state, as well as by hormones and alcohol.
  - ○ activates vitamins (thiamine, pyridoxine, folic acid, vitamin D). It also synthesises carrier proteins for vitamins, such as A and B_{12} and lipoproteins to transport vitamin E. Furthermore, liver stores vitamins A, D, E, K and B_{12}.
  - ○ stores copper, iron and zinc.

What is the dietary treatment for acute hepatitis?

Regardless of cause, acute liver injury is often associated with anorexia, nausea and vomiting. Thus, acute liver injury is likely to decrease the oral intake of food, but if the illness is short-lived, nutritional consequences are minimal. Both alcoholic and non-alcoholic acute liver injury may cause fasting hypoglycaemia. This has been attributed to depleted liver glycogen reserves and a block in gluconeogenesis from amino acids.

Chapter 7

Nutritional management during the acute phase aims at providing adequate amounts of energy, macro- and micronutrients for the regeneration of hepatocytes. In this phase, energy and protein needs are increased; however, diets with excessive energy and protein should be avoided. Patients with viral acute hepatitis should be administered a healthy balanced diet, with a small increase in protein intake [1.2–1.5 g/kg (2.64–3.3 g/lb) body weight]. Severe reductions in fat intake should be avoided since low-fat diets are unpalatable and may enhance a patient's anorexia and undernutrition. Small and frequent meals are generally better tolerated. If anorexia, nausea and vomiting persist, fluid and/or nutrient needs should be administered by enteral or parenteral nutrition. During the acute phase as well as for the next six months, the patient should completely abstain from alcohol consumption, because of its hepatotoxicity.

Patients with fulminant hepatitis may experience severe episodes of hypoglycaemia, caused by reduced glycogen stores and impaired glyconeogenesis. Moreover, they may develop severe malnutrition because of excessive nitrogen loss that follows massive liver necrosis. In this case, stabilisation of metabolism is mandatory and more important than nutritional therapy, and should aim to meet daily requirements. According to guidelines provided by the European Society for Clinical Nutrition and Metabolism (ESPEN), these patients need stable glucose administration (150–200 g), often given parenterally through dextrose solutions. In the case of enteral nutrition, patients should receive it via a nasoduodenal tube; however, no recommendations concerning the type of formula are currently available. Excessive protein administration should be avoided because it may precipitate hepatic encephalopathy. Owing to severe liver failure, glucose, lactate, triglycerides and ammonia plasma levels should be closely monitored and used as surrogate markers of substrate utilisation.

What is non-alcoholic fatty liver disease and what is its dietary treatment?

Non-alcoholic fatty liver disease (NAFLD) represents a spectrum of hepatic disorders characterised by macrovesicular steatosis that occur in the absence of alcohol consumption or with intakes generally considered not harmful to the liver (less than 40 g of ethanol per day). That spectrum ranges from simple hepatic steatosis (most usual case) without concomitant inflammation or fibrosis to hepatic steatosis with a necroinflammatory component that may or may not have associated fibrosis (non-alcoholic steatohepatitis, or NASH) and can progress to cryptogenic cirrhosis. There is increasing evidence that NAFLD represents the hepatic component of the metabolic syndrome characterised by central obesity, hyperinsulinaemia, peripheral insulin resistance, diabetes, hypertriglyceridaemia and hypertension.

Obesity, particularly central obesity, is strongly associated with hepatic steatosis. For this reason, lifestyle modification that includes dietary restriction and exercise to achieve judicious weight loss, in addition to the control of risk factors such as type 2 diabetes mellitus, obesity, dyslipidaemia and oxidative stress, is recommended as the cornerstone of treatment and prevention of NAFLD. Little is known about the effects of changes in dietary composition on liver histopathology in NAFLD, since few studies have addressed this issue and for this reason the best dietary approach for the treatment of NAFLD has not been established by experimental evidence. In the absence of such evidence, approaches used for diabetes and 'heart healthy' dietary composition seem prudent. Short-term weight loss with concomitant exercise leads to an improvement in liver biochemical tests and to the resolution of hepatic steatosis. Moderate weight loss with incorporated regular physical activity ($\geq$20 min aerobic exercise) is advocated in contrast to rapid weigh loss, which could aggravate the underlying liver disease. The dietary treatment includes some caloric restriction, a diet low in saturated fats with relative enrichment of unsaturated fats, and one low in rapidly absorbable carbohydrates (high glycaemic index), but high in slowly absorbable carbohydrates (especially those high in dietary fibre) and alcohol abstinence. Some investigators have proposed that antioxidant supplements may be useful for NAFLD treatment; however, there is insufficient data to either support or refute the use of antioxidant supplements in these patients and large prospective randomised clinical trials on this topic are required.

What are the most common cholestatic syndromes and what dietary modifications do they require?

Primary biliary sclerosis and primary sclerosing cholangitis are two syndromes accompanied with cholestasis. Patients with these conditions usually suffer from chronic fat malabsorption and subsequent steatorrhoea, which leads to significant losses of fluids and electrolytes, as well as to deterioration of the nutritional status. In these cases severe fat restriction is necessary (low-fat diet: 40–50 g of fat or very low-fat diet: 25–30 g of fat) with the adequate administration of energy and proteins. Fat distribution throughout the day and MCT administration may help patients with severe symptoms. High oxalic acid intake, as well as that of ascorbic acid should be avoided for the prevention of renal stones formation. Calcium intake should be as high as 1500 mg/day and in the event of supplement intake; this should take place between meals. The frequent monitoring of plasma fat-soluble vitamins is necessary, since deficiencies are quite common. Oftentimes, patients with chronic cholestasis present hyperlipidaemias which are, however, not associated with atherogenesis, and for this reason dietary interventions for the treatment of these conditions are not necessary.

What are the main causes of malnutrition in end-stage liver disease?

The cause of malnutrition among patients with end-stage liver disease (ESLD) is multifactorial. Nutritional status is influenced mainly by:

- inadequacy of dietary intake due to anorexia, dysgeusia, nausea and feeling of fullness which are caused by ascites, jaundice, infections, delayed gastric emptying and drug therapy or even by reduced activity of these

Chapter 7

patients. Moreover, other factors resulting in inadequate dietary intake are the unpalatable diets often prescribed to ESLD patients or heavy alcoholism, as well as the reduced levels of consciousness or reduced food intake, due to increased alcohol consumption

- nutrient maldigestion and malabsorption owing to reduced bile acids secretion or to concurrent pancreatic insufficiency, chronic pancreatitis, alcohol toxicity and, in some cases, enteropathies
- negative nitrogen balance owing to increased protein degradation for the purposes of glyconeogenesis, decreased protein synthesis caused by liver impairment and increased protein losses mainly caused by common complications of ESLD, such as ascites, renal dysfunction and intestinal bleeding
- altered nutrient metabolism and substrate utilisation
- increased energy expenditure, although not present in all ESLD patients
- psychosocial factors.

On what information should the nutritional assessment of a patient with end-stage liver disease focus?

Objective parameters of nutritional assessment are not always valid in patients with ESLD since most of the common markers of nutritional assessment are influenced by liver diseases. During nutritional assessment, the dietitian should focus on:

- the history, severity, duration and cause of liver disease, as well as on the concurrent diseases (e.g. renal dysfunction, heart or pancreatic failure, diabetes mellitus) and medication, which can affect dietary intake and nutritional status in many ways
- signs and symptoms related to ESLD complications, such as alterations in conscious level, presence of jaundice, ascites, oedema or bruises, especially in the lower parts of the body, signs of nutritional inadequacy (e.g. zinc deficiency acrodermatitis, pellagra due to niacin deficiency, etc.), skin scratches due to steatorrhoea causing itching
- history of body weight, since recent weight loss may reflect negative energy balance. However, in many ESLD patients body weight cannot offer information on nutritional status since it is significantly affected by fluid retention (e.g. in ascites and oedema)
- anthropometric indices of the upper part of the body, namely triceps skinfold (TSF), mid-arm circumference (MAC) and mid-arm muscle circumference (MAMC), since they are slightly influenced by fluid retention and give quite reliable estimations of nutritional status. Reduced MAC values usually reflect a general weight loss, reduced TSF values correspond to severe losses of fat deposits, whereas reduced MAMC values reflect severe protein losses and exhaustion of protein deposits
- detailed dietary history for the assessment of dietary intake, potential nutrient deficiencies or alcohol intake, in order to decide whether nutritional support should be initiated.

Furthermore, health professionals should bear in mind that classical indices of nutritional status such as plasma albumin, prealbumin, transferrin or retinol-binding protein cannot offer valid estimation of nutritional status in ESLD patients since they are reduced due to liver failure, renal impairment and/or fluid retention.

What are the main complications of liver cirrhosis? Do they require any special nutritional management?

Table 7.5 summarises the most common complications of ESLD and the main dietary treatment for these conditions.

Are there any specific nutritional concerns during the pre-operative period of liver transplantation?

Patients who are scheduled to undergo liver transplantation should be of a good nutritional status since malnutrition has been shown to adversely affect post-transplant outcomes. During the pre-transplant period, patients should receive 30 kcal/kg of desired body weight (1.2–1.3 × basal metabolic rate, based on the Harris-Benedict equation, see Chapter 2) and 0.8–1.2 g/kg (1.76–2.64 g/lb) dry body weight of protein, if weight preservation is the main aim. Moreover, some patients with ESLD may experience hypoglycaemic episodes, and in these patients a stable administration of 150–200 g of carbohydrates throughout the day is crucial, either through diet or parenterally with dextrose solutions. Transplant candidates with malnutrition should receive 35–40 kcal/kg (322–368 kJ/lb) dry body weight (or 1.5 × basal metabolic rate) and 1.3 – 2 g protein/kg (2.86–4.4 g/lb) dry body weight for repletion. Calories and nutrients should be preferably administered orally, distributed in 4–7 meals and snacks, and fasting periods longer than six hours should be avoided. When food intake does not reach the desired goals, enteral nutrition may be administered in combination with food. Apart from malnutrition, obesity has been hypothesised to adversely affect post-transplant recovery. Obese transplant candidates should receive dietary advice for weight control.

What is the dietary regime for liver recipients during the short- and long-term post-transplant period?

The first two months after liver transplantation require special dietary management. During this phase, a patient should receive 30–35 kcal/kg (276–322 kJ/lb) of dry or desired body weight (or 120–140% of basal metabolic rate, based on the Harris-Benedict equation, see Chapter 2). Protein intake should range between 1.2 and 1.7 g/kg (2.64–3.74 g/lb) dry body weight; however, in the event of renal insufficiency this should be reduced to 1.2–1.5 g/kg (2.64–3.3 g/lb). Carbohydrates should cover 50–70% of non-protein calories and simple carbohydrates should be avoided, especially during corticosteroid use. Optimal fluid intake should be equal to 30–35 ml/kg

Chapter 7

Table 7.5 Common dietary treatment of end-stage liver disease complications.

Complication	Dietary management
Ascites	Add 10% as a stress factor when calculating energy needs.
	Protein intake around 1.2–1.5 g/kg BW[a]
	Limit sodium intake to 2000 mg per day. Avoid further reduction, because this leads to unpalatable diets and risk of malnutrition.
	Fluid restriction is necessary only in cases of severe plasma hyponatraemia (<120 mmol/l), in parallel with sodium restriction and diuretics administration.
	Careful monitoring of potassium. Possible hyperkalaemia or hypokalaemia due to diuretics.
Encephalopathy	Limit protein intake to 0.6–0.8 g/kg BW (especially in stages III and IV) until the cause of encephalopathy is treated properly (e.g. bleeding, infection, electrolyte imbalance, sedatives, constipation). Then gradually increase intake up to 1.2–1.5 g/kg BW.
	If encephalopathy persists, try 0.6 g protein/BW and a supplement of branched-chain amino acids (BCAA).
	Provide adequate energy (25–35 kcal/kg BW) to attenuate protein degradation.
	Give dietary advice that helps preventing/treating constipation, apart from medication.
	Administer zinc supplement if zinc deficiency is suspected.
Cholestasis/steatorrhoea	Ensure adequate energy (35–45 kcal/kg BW or 1.5–1.75 × basal energy expenditure) and protein (1.2–1.5 g/kg BW) intake.
	Administer a low- or very low-fat diet. If diarrhoea does not resolve, discontinue fat restriction.
	Try medium-chain triglycerides.
	Careful monitoring of fat-soluble vitamins.
Malnutrition	Provide 35–45 kcal/kg BW or at least 120% of estimated energy expenditure.
	Provide 1.2–1.8 g of protein/kg BW.
	Try small, frequent, energy-dense meals/snacks. Consider providing an oral supplement.
	Carbohydrate intake: 50–55% of daily calories, fat intake: 30–35% of daily calories.

[a] BW: body weight. In overweight or obese subjects, use desired or adjusted body weight. For patients with fluid retention, estimate a dry body weight or use a desired body weight for the calculations. Finally, use current or usual body weight for patients without fluid retention and within the normal ranges of body mass index.

Chapter 7

(2.32–2.7 fl oz/lb) body weight. Oral diet is usually initiated when the patient is passing flatus. Start with a clear liquid diet for the first 1–2 meals and quickly advance to the above-mentioned regimen. Enteral nutrition may be necessary for the first post-transplant days if the patient will not receive adequate oral nutrition, whereas parenteral nutrition is indicated in cases of a non-functioning gut (e.g. ileus).

During the long-term post-transplant period caloric needs range from 30 to 35 kcal/kg (276–322 kJ/lb) body weight (or 1.2–1.3 × basal metabolic rate) and protein intake should be reduced to 0.8–1.0 g/kg (1.76–2.2 g/lb). During corticosteroid administration, protein needs may be slightly higher. With regard to carbohydrates and fat intake, these should follow the guidelines of a healthy diet for adults. During corticosteroid use, calcium intake should be at 1200–1500 mg per day and, owing to immunosuppressant agents, patients should avoid grapefruit intake and handle food carefully to avoid food-borne illnesses. Patients should also abstain from alcohol consumption and during this period they may also experience excessive weight gain, hyperlipidaemia, diabetes mellitus or osteoporosis, which require special nutritional therapies.

What dietary modifications are needed in cholelithiasis and cholecystitis?

Individuals with gallstones should modify their diet until they undergo a cholecystectomy. In general a dietary fat restriction is indicated in these patients; however, there is no strong scientific evidence to necessitate severe fat restriction (e.g. <40 g/day). Oftentimes, patients with gallstones experience unpleasant symptoms after the ingestion of certain foods, especially legumes and large quantities of raw, leafy vegetables and in that case a reduction in these foods' consumption may alleviate symptoms. Increased fluid intake especially in the form of water is also very important for these patients.

In the case of acute cholecystitis the patient should need hospitalisation for some days and during the first 24 hours discontinuation of oral nutrition is necessary and patients should receive fluids and electrolytes parenterally. When oral intake is initiated, a liquid diet and then progression to a very low-fat diet (25–30 g of fat) will help keep gallbladder stimulation relatively low. If this diet is well tolerated, then a low-fat diet (45–50 g of fat) should be introduced. Moreover, fibres should be also gradually introduced so that the patient can identify the amount of fibres that they can tolerate. The above-mentioned dietary advice should be indicated during the first weeks after cholecystectomy, although with the passage of time these patients will receive a normal, unrestricted, diet.

What are the main causes of acute pancreatitis and how is the stage of its severity estimated?

Among the most common causes of acute pancreatitis belong gallstones (including microlithiasis), alcohol consumption/abuse, hyperlipidaemia, drugs and toxins intake, as well as trauma in the region of the abdomen and post-operative complications. The diagnostic process of acute pancreatitis is based on the clinician's index of suspicion; this index is formed by taking a clinical history and then examining the patient in order to determine the so-called pretest probability of disease. Whenever acute upper abdominal pain is combined with elevated pancreatic enzyme levels, the final diagnosis will be fully established by imaging and/or the manner in which the clinical course of the disease unfolds. The mortality of acute pancreatitis is dependent on a number of factors, including the age and obesity of the patient. Up to 50% of patients who die may do so within the first seven days of illness, from multiple organ dysfunction syndrome (MODS). Multifactorial grading systems are usually applied to assess acute pancreatitis' severity, such as APACHE II and the Glasgow or Ranson scoring systems, and to categorise it as either mild, moderate or severe.

What dietary protocol should be followed in mild or moderate acute pancreatitis?

Acute pancreatitis is a hypercatabolic state resulting in the rapid loss of body weight, fat and protein. Nutritional support is an integral part of patient care and is started early in the course of the disease. Patients with mild to moderate disease (80% of patients) will receive supportive care for several days, including pain control, intravenous fluids and nil by mouth. Because most patients eat within 5–7 days of presentation, they do not require specialised nutritional support, such as jejunal or parenteral nutrition. Feeding these patients usually begins by giving 100–300 ml (3.5–10.55 fl oz) of liquids, containing no calories, every four hours for the first 24 hours. Clear liquid diets have no fat and therefore present less risk of pancreatic stimulation as initial feeding. If this diet is tolerated, oral feeding is advanced to giving the same volume of liquids containing low-fat nutrients. Subsequently, if patients continue to do well, feedings are changed gradually over 3–4 days to soft and finally solid foods. All the diets contain greater than 50% of calories in the form of carbohydrate, are moderate in protein [1.2–1.5 g/kg (2.64–3.3 g/lb) body weight] and fat [starting from 0.8 g/kg (2.64 g/lb) body weight] and the total caloric content is gradually increased from 160 to 640 kcal (670–2680 kJ) per meal. Before stepping to a normal diet, a low-fat diet may be useful for a short period for patients recovering from pancreatitis.

What route of nutritional support is recommended for patients with severe acute pancreatitis?

In patients with severe acute pancreatitis either total parenteral nutrition (TPN) or enteral nutrition (EN) is employed. TPN is effective in preventing protein catabolism and also 'rests' the pancreas, but increases the already high risk of septic and metabolic side effects and may worsen the outcome in mild illness. EN should be initiated as early as possible, particularly when alcoholism, with its associated undernutrition, is the cause. Water, electrolyte and micronutrient requirements must be met by the intravenous route and decreased gradually as the enteral supply increases. The most likely reason for the superiority of EN over TPN is its capacity to maintain intestinal function, maintaining intestinal integrity and the gut mucosal barrier, which may in turn decrease the risk of bacterial translocation and subsequent septic complications. Moreover, it can suppress the cytokine-mediated systemic inflammatory response and consequent multiple organ failure.

The leading groups in the UK and continental Europe now employ early EN in preference to intravenous feeding in patients with severe acute pancreatitis, swinging towards the early use of naso-enteric feeding with a lowering of the risk associated with TPN. The European Society for Clinical Nutrition and Metabolism's (ESPEN) guidelines on enteral nutrition in acute pancreatitis suggest the jejunal route if gastric feeding is not tolerated. Generally, the more distally a tube is placed in the small bowel, the less pancreatic stimulation occurs. In the event of surgery for pancreatitis an intraoperative jejunostomy for postoperative tube feeding is recommended. The placement of a jejunostomy tube beyond the ligament of Treitz, coupled with the slow continuous infusion of an enteral formula, results in almost no pancreatic stimulation and offers considerable advantages over TPN. In gastric outlet obstruction, the tube tip should be placed distal to the obstruction. If this is impossible, parenteral nutrition should be given. Tube feeding is also possible in the presence of ascites and pancreatic fistulas.

With regard to type of enteral formula, most trials (human and animal) have been carried out using peptide-based feedings. Whether standard formulas can be used safely or immune-modulating formulas have an additional impact on the course of the disease remains unclear. Today it is common to start with a standard formula and if this is not tolerated a peptide-based one is tried. If enteral nutrition is not tolerated, parenteral nutrition is required. The preferred solution contains carbohydrate, protein and lipid. The exception to this is hypertriglyceridaemia (one of the main causes of acute pancreatitis), in which case lipid should be excluded. Both in the case of EN and TPN if fat is administered, serum triglycerides should be monitored regularly. Values below 10–12 mmol/l are tolerated but serum lipid levels should ideally be kept within normal ranges.

Septic complications are important causes of increased resting energy expenditure. A patient's individual caloric requirement can be calculated by using the Harris-Benedict equation (see Chapter 2) with appropriate modifications for stress factors, although objections have been expressed concerning their accuracy. Otherwise, 25–35 kcal/kg (230–322 kJ/lb) body weight is an acceptable range of energy requirements and the use of indirect calorimetry can also give accurate estimates. In general, patients with severe acute pancreatitis will require 1.2–1.5 g/kg (2.64–3.3 g/lb) body weight of protein. Carbohydrates should range between 3 and 6 g/kg (6.6–13.2 g/lb) corresponding to blood glucose concentration, which values should be <10 mmol/l and lipids intake up to 2 g/kg (4.4 g/lb), beginning usually from 0.8 g/kg (1.76 g/lb) and always according to triglyceride concentration.

Chapter 7

What is the dietary approach for patients with chronic pancreatitis?

Protein energy malnutrition is a common finding in patients with chronic pancreatitis and its causes are multifactorial, including the recurrent pain following meals (sitophobia), steatorrhoea, anorexia, nausea, diarrhoea and oftentimes concurrent alcoholism. Moreover, many patients also have diabetes, which contributes to anorexia and weight loss. Although energy requirements may be increased by 15 to 30% of what is expected based on the Harris-Benedict equation, excessive overfeeding should be avoided. Ideally, the patient should be maintained in a positive nitrogen balance by feeding total calories based on the Harris-Benedict equation plus 20%, which equates approximately to 25–30 kcal/kg/day (230–276 kJ/lb/day). Protein should supply approximately 1.0 to 1.5 g/kg/day (2.2–3.3 g/lb/day) and lipids should comprise approximately 30% of the total calories, depending on the symptoms of each patient (pain, steatorrhoea). Patients experiencing intense symptoms usually benefit from further fat restriction (i.e. 40–60 g per day). In this case, MCTs may be also administered to cover some of the calories required. Carbohydrates should cover 40–60% of the daily calories; however, hyperglycaemia may occur, and insulin may be required to maintain a serum glucose concentration between normal range. Total abstinence from alcohol is also required, and treatment of exocrine insufficiency relies on pancreatic enzyme replacement, which is administered during mealtimes. In patients with severe steatorrhoea, fat-soluble vitamins should be closely monitored. Moreover, the replacement of combined antioxidants (selenium, methionine, vitamins A, C and E) has been shown to reduce pancreatic inflammation and pain in patients with both acute and chronic pancreatitis. Small studies have suggested that daily antioxidants should include 600 μg of organic selenium, 9000 IU of vitamin A, 500 mg of vitamin C, 270 IU of vitamin E, and 2 g of methionine.

Chapter 7

Further reading

Akobeng AK (2008) Review article: The evidence base for interventions used to maintain remission in Crohn's disease. *Alimentary Pharmacology and Theraputics* **27**(1): 11–18.

Alvarez-Leite JL (2004) Nutrient deficiencies secondary to bariatric surgery. *Current Opinion in Clinical Nutrition and Metabolic Care* **7**: 569–75.

American College of Gastroenterology Task Force on Irritable Bowel Syndrome, Brandt LJ, Chey WD *et al.* (2009) An evidence-based position statement on the management of irritable bowel syndrome. *American Journal of Gastroenterology* **104**(suppl. 1): S1–35.

Brownlee HJ (1990) Family practitioner's guide to patient self-treatment of acute diarrhea. *American Journal of Medicine* **88**(suppl. 6A): S27–9.

Chan HL, de Silva HJ, Leung NW *et al.* (2007) How should we manage patients with non-alcoholic fatty liver disease in 2007? *Journal of Gastroenterology and Hepatology* **22**: 801–8.

Craig D, Robins G, Howdle PD (2007) Advances in celiac disease. *Current Opinion in Gastroenterology* **23**(2): 142–8.

DiBaise JK (2008) Management of the short bowel syndrome. In: *Nutrition and Gastrointestinal Disease*, DeLegge MH (ed.), Humana Press Inc., Totowa, NJ.

Dietitians of Canada (2003) Hepatitis C: Nutrition care. *Canadian Guidelines for Health Care Providers*, http://www.dietitians.ca/resources/resourcesearch. asp?fn=view&contentid=2516.

Fox M, Barr C, Nolan S *et al.* (2007) The effects of dietary fat and calorie density on esophageal acid exposure and reflux symptoms. *Clinical Gastroenterology Hepatology* **5**(4): 439–44.

Garsed K, Scott BB (2007) Can oats be taken in a gluten-free diet? A systematic review. *Scandinavian Journal of Gastroenterology*, **42**(2): 171–8.

Green PHR, Cellier C (2007) Celiac Disease. *New England Journal of Medicine* **357**: 1731–43.

Heizer WD, Southern S, McGovern S (2009) The role of diet in symptoms of irritable bowel syndrome in adults: A narrative review. *Journal of the American Dietetic Association* **109**(7): 1204–14.

Lacy BE, Weiser K (2008) Esophageal motility disorders: Medical therapy. *Journal of Clinical Gastroenterology* **42**(5): 652–8.

MacLean CH, Mojica WA, Newberry SJ *et al.* (2005) Systematic review of the effects of omega-3 fatty acids in inflammatory bowel disease. *American Journal of Clinical Nutrition* **82**(3): 611–9.

Mathew P, Wyllie R, Van Lente F *et al.* (1996) Antioxidants in hereditary pancreatitis. *American Journal of Gastroenterology* **91**(8): 1558–62.

Meier R, Beglinger C, Layer P *et al.* (2002) ESPEN guidelines on nutrition in acute pancreatitis. *Clinical Nutrition* **21**(2): 173–83.

Meier R, Ockenga J, Pertkiewicz M *et al.* (2006) ESPEN guidelines on enteral nutrition: Pancreas. *Clinical Nutrition* **25**(2): 275–84.

Meining A, Classen M (2000) The role of diet and lifestyle measures in the pathogenesis and treatment of gastroesophageal reflux disease. *American Journal of Gastroenterology* **95**(10): 2692–7.

Parker TJ, Naylor SJ, Riordan AM, Hunter JO (1995) Management of patients with food intolerance in irritable bowel syndrome: The development and use of an exclusion diet. *Journal of Human Nutrition and Dietetics* **8**: 159–66.

Plautha M, Cabre E, Riggio O *et al.* (2006) ESPEN guidelines on enteral nutrition: Liver disease. *Clinical Nutrition* **25**: 285–94.

Ryan-Harshman M, Aldoori W (2004) How diet and lifestyle affect duodenal ulcers: Review of the evidence. *Canadian Family Physician* **50**: 727–32.

Sheil B, Shanahan F, O'Mahony L (2007) Probiotic effects on inflammatory bowel disease. *Journal of Nutrition* **137**(3, suppl. 2): S819–24.

Toouli J, Brooke-Smith M, Bassi C *et al.* (2002) Guidelines for the management of acute pancreatitis. *Journal of Gastroenterology and Hepatology* **17**(suppl.): S15–39.

Van Gossum A, Closset P, Noel E *et al.* (1996) Deficiency in antioxidant factors in patients with alcohol-related chronic pancreatitis. *Digestive Diseases and Sciences* **41**(6): 1225–31.

Watts GF, Gan SK (2008) Nutrition and metabolism: Non-alcoholic fatty liver disease: Pathogenesis, cardiovascular risk and therapy. *Current Opinion in Lipidology* **19**: 92–4.

Chapter 7

Wild GE, Drozdowski L, Tartaglia C *et al.* (2007) Nutritional modulation of the inflammatory response in inflammatory bowel disease: From the molecular to the integrative to the clinical. *World Journal of Gastroenterology* **13**(1): 1–7.

Wilmore DW, Robinson MK (2000) Short bowel syndrome. *World Journal of Surgery* **24**(12): 1486–92.

Chapter 8

Renal Disease

Kalliopi-Anna Poulia

What are the main components of nephrotic syndrome?

Nephrotic syndrome is the condition resulting from loss of the glomerular barrier to protein, characterised by:

- excess albuminuria ($>3.0\,g/24\,hr$)
- hypoalbuminaemia
- massive peripheral oedema
- hyperlipidaemia
- hypertension.

What are the dietary needs of patients with nephrotic syndrome?

The main goals of medical nutrition therapy in patients with nephrotic syndrome are the reduction of protein losses in urine, the provision of sufficient energy, to prevent malnutrition and the prevention of the evolution of nephrotic syndrome to chronic renal failure.

In the past, high-protein diets were advocated for these patients. However, those diets proved to be inappropriate, as they could increase albuminuria. Current recommendations suggest a moderate protein intake of $0.8\,g/kg$ ideal body weight (IBW) per day, with close monitoring for malnutrition, and if needed dietary protein intake can increase up to $1.0\,g/kg$ IBW. These protein intakes have been proven to raise serum albumin levels, with no adverse effects on albuminuria. Moreover, sodium restriction to less than $6\,g/day$ is also necessary, in order to minimise oedema and hypertension and to potentiate the effect of angiotensin-converting enzyme (ACE) inhibitors and angiotensin receptor blockers (ARBs). Regarding hyperlipidaemia in these patients, the dietary treatment alone is usually not sufficient. Despite the fact that dietary treatment of hyperlipidaemia in nephrotic syndrome has not been fully investigated, low-fat, low-cholesterol, high-complex-carbohydrate diets, adjusted for the individual's energy and protein needs, should be prescribed.

Should patients with renal stones follow a special diet?

Renal stones are generally generated when the concentration of components in the urine is above the level that allows crystallisation. According to their chemical constituents, they are classified as:

- calcium stones
- uric acid stones
- cystine stones
- struvite stones.

Regardless of the type of renal stone, patients should be encouraged to increase their fluid intake in order to produce at least two litres of urine per day. Moreover, sodium restriction seems to be beneficial for patients with renal stones, as urinary sodium excretion is correlated with calcium, uric acid and cystine excretion.

In the past, patients with calcium stones were advised to reduce calcium intake. However, calcium restriction (<400 mg/day) does not positively affect calcium stone formation. On the contrary, the reduction of dietary oxalate is advised, as the majority of urinary calculi contain oxalate. The principal dietary sources of oxalate are spinach, beetroots, strawberries, chocolate, peanuts, tea and rhubarb. Moreover, as vitamin C is important for the formation of oxalic acid in the human body, the supplemental intake of this vitamin should be avoided [reference nutrient intake (RNI) = 60 mg/day, recommended dietary allowance (RDA) = 60–95 mg/day].

Regarding uric acid stones, patients should be advised to decrease their protein intake, especially from sources with a high purine content. In addition to that, other dietary sources of purine should be avoided. (See Chapter 14's section on gout.)

What are the types of acute renal failure?

Acute renal failure (ARF) is a condition characterised by the sudden reduction in the glomerular filtration rate (GFR) and an alteration in the kidney's ability to excrete metabolic wastes, leading to uraemia, metabolic acidosis, and fluid and electrolytic imbalances. Typically, it occurs in previously healthy kidneys and can be caused by:

- inadequate renal perfusion (pre-renal ARF)
- diseases within the kidney (intrinsic ARF), mainly due to nephrotoxic drugs
- obstruction, often due to renal tumours or renal stones (post-renal ARF).

What are the energy and protein needs in acute renal failure?

The management of patients with ARF is rather complicated owing to uraemia, metabolic acidosis, and fluid and electrolytic imbalances, in combination with physiological stress from the underlying cause of ARF.

Table 8.1 Classification of chronic kidney disease.

Stage	Description	eGFR (ml/min/1.73m^2)
1	Kidney damage with normal or elevated eGFR	$\geq$90
2	Kidney damage with mild reduction of eGFR	60–89
3	Moderate reduction of eGFR	30–59
4	Severe reduction of eGFR	15–29
5	Kidney failure	<15 (or dialysis)

eGFR = estimated glomerular filtration rate.

Therefore, balancing the high protein and energy needs with the need for limiting the demand on the kidney for the excretion of nitrogen is a very delicate operation.

These patients' energy needs vary greatly, depending on the underlying cause of the ARF and any comorbidity. Ideally, energy needs should be assessed by indirect calorimetry. In clinical settings in which this measurement is not often possible, the provision of 30–40 kcal/kg IBW seems to be sufficient for the majority of the patients. When in the early stages of ARF, patients are likely to be anorexic and unable to tolerate oral nutrition, owing to vomiting and diarrhoea. In this case, total parenteral nutrition (TPN) may be considered, in order to reduce protein catabolism. Regarding the dietary protein intake, the recommendations suggest a protein intake ranging from 0.6–0.8 g/kg IBW for non-dialysed patients to 1.0–2.0 g/kg IBW for those undergoing dialysis. As patients stabilise, it is agreed that protein intake should be 0.8–1.0 g/kg.

What are the stages of chronic kidney disease?

Patients with chronic kidney disease (CKD), irrespective of diagnosis, are classified according to the Kidney Disease Outcomes Quality Initiative guidelines of the National Kidney Foundation (NKF KDOQI) CKD classification (Table 8.1).

What are the main goals of nutritional care in chronic kidney disease?

The main aims of nutritional therapy in CKD are:

- to maintain good nutritional status, through adequate macro- and micronutrient intake
- to control the symptoms and minimise metabolic disorders (oedema, hypoalbuminaemia and hyperlipidaemia)
- to retard the progress of CKD to renal failure and the necessity for dialysis

Chapter 8

- to prevent or delay the development of renal osteodystrophy, by controlling phosphorus, calcium and vitamin D intake
- the provision of a palatable and attractive diet plan, which reflects the patient's lifestyle and needs.

What factors contribute to malnutrition in patients with chronic kidney disease?

Epidemiological studies have reported a significant low energy intake in end-stage renal patients, reaching as much as 20–25 kcal/kg/day, owing to reduced appetite and uraemia-induced gastrointestinal disturbances. Despite the caloric intake by the dextrose in the dialysate, malnutrition is also common in peritoneal dialysis (PD) patients, owing to the feeling of fullness that the dialysate causes to the patient, the loss of appetite and/or the increased energy needs precipitated by peritonitis.

How are the energy and protein needs of adult patients with chronic kidney disease calculated?

The evaluation of the energy needs in renal patients is vital, as sufficient energy intake can contribute to the maintenance of a body weight within the normal range for body mass index (BMI) and to the achievement of a positive nitrogen balance.

According to recent recommendations, the provision of 35 kcal/kg IBW is sufficient for the majority of pre-dialysis renal patients. Lower energy intake (i.e. 30–35 kcal/kg/day) is recommended for patients >60 years old or for patients with a sedentary way of life.

For the prevention of energy/protein malnutrition in clinically stable chronic haemodialysis patients, energy intake should be 30–35 kcal/kg/day, adjusted for age, gender and physical activity levels. For patients undergoing peritoneal dialysis, calories absorbed from the dialysate should be included in the assessment of the nutritional needs of the patients. Sixty to seventy per cent of the dextrose of the dialysate is absorbed during its stay in the peritoneal cavity. Therefore, the energy intake for PD patients should be 30–35 kcal/kg IBW/day, including the calories for the dialysate.

What are the recommendations for sodium, phosphorus and calcium, and potassium intake in adult patients with chronic kidney disease?

Sodium

Sodium as an extracellular electrolyte facilitates the regulation of fluid balance. Restriction of sodium to the level 'no added salt' should be implemented in patients with oedemas or hypertension. In end-stage CKD, as urine output decreases, sodium filtration decreases as well and sodium intake should be limited to 2000–2300 mg/day (80–100 mmol). Sodium restriction in these patients contributes to better fluid intake control through lowering thirst sensation. However, if the patient is dehydrated, sodium intake must be temporarily increased.

Phosphorus and calcium

Hyperphosphataemia is a common problem in patients in the late stages of CKD. Phosphorus retention is directly connected to the development of secondary hyperparathyroidism, leading to renal osteodystrophy. According to the NKF KDOQI guidelines, serum phosphate should be kept within the range of 2.7 to 4.6 mg/d (0.87–1.49 mmol/l) in patients with GFR between 15 and 59 ml/min (stage 3 and 4 patients). Whereas for patients with CKD stage 5 and on dialysis the serum phosphate level should be 1.1–1.8 mmol/l. In the event of abnormal laboratory values of serum phosphate, dietary phosphorus intake should be limited. It should be stressed, though, that the restriction in phosphorus is easy to achieve in patients with limited protein intake, as they are advised to limit their intake of the main dietary sources of this mineral (i.e. dairy products, meat and animal protein). In contrast, when patients commence dialysis, dietary phosphate restriction is more of a challenge as protein requirements are increased. According to the NKF KDOQI and European guidelines, phosphate intake should be limited to 800–1000 mg/day. High-protein foods with a lower phosphate content should be recommended, to ensure lower phosphate intake without lowering the protein intake, in combination with non-dietary strategies (i.e. phosphate binders and optimum dialysis prescriptions).

An imbalance of phosphorus and calcium can increase soft tissue and vascular calcification, leading to higher cardiovascular disease prevalence and mortality in patients with CKD stage 3 to 5. Therefore, the current KDOQI guidelines focus on the balance between phosphate and calcium. More specifically, the calcium phosphate product (corrected calcium × phosphate) should be <4.4 mmol^2/l^2 in these patients.

As for dietary calcium intake in CKD patients, it should not exceed 2000 mg daily; this includes calcium obtained from calcium-based phosphate binders for the management of renal bone disease and metabolism.

Potassium

Hyperkalaemia is common in patients with advanced kidney disease (stage 4 to 5 CKD), raising their risk of sudden cardiac death. Renal insufficiency, metabolic acidosis, lean body mass catabolism and insufficient dialysis are some of the causes of hyperkalaemia in these patients. Moreover, medical therapies such as ACE inhibitors, ARB, beta-blockers, potassium

Chapter 8

sparing diuretics, non-steroidal anti-inflammatory drugs, corticosteroids and cyclosporine use can also raise potassium blood levels.

In the early stages of CKD, serum potassium levels are usually within the normal values, whereas with patients at stages 3 to 5, serum potassium should be monitored and their potassium intake restricted when a rising trend in serum potassium levels is observed or when hyperkalaemia occurs (i.e. >5.5 mmol/l). Elevated serum potassium levels for dialysis patients are defined as >6 mmol/l. Dietary potassium intake should be limited to 51–77 mmol/2000–3000 mg/day (8–17 mg or 1 mmol/kg/kg IBW/day).

Normal bowel function can also contribute to normal serum potassium values. In order to compensate for renal insufficiency, the large intestine increases stool potassium content. Therefore, the prevention of constipation can help in achieving normal serum potassium levels.

What are the vitamin and trace element needs of patients with chronic kidney disease? Should they be altered, according to the stage of the renal failure?

Vitamin and mineral requirements are still a controversial issue in CKD patients. Renal patients may be in danger of vitamin deficiencies due to compromised dietary intake and/or appetite, dietary restrictions leading to insufficient intake of nutrients, the process of haemodialysis and PD that raises water-soluble vitamin losses and other pathological problems that could increase patients' needs.

Supplementation of water-soluble vitamins should be considered in patients with compromised dietary intake. Folic acid supplementation of 1 mg/day should be used for the prevention of megaloblastic anaemia. Higher doses of 5 mg/day are suggested for the treatment of hyperhomocysteinaemia and the protection of cardiovascular disease. Vitamin C supplements should not exceed 75–90 mg/day, as intakes higher than 100 mg/day are implicated in the formation of oxalate renal stones.

Regarding the supplementation of lipid-soluble vitamins, patients with CKD are usually prescribed with analogues of vitamin D, to prevent renal osteodystrophy. Vitamin A and K supplementation should be avoided because of the danger of toxicity in these patients. As for vitamin E intake, recent European guidelines suggest a supplemental intake of 400–800 IU for the secondary prevention of cardiovascular events and recurrent muscle cramps.

Mineral supplementation, including trace element supplementation, should be done with great caution. Iron supplementation should be individualised to patients' needs and monitored closely. The supplemental use of iron should be considered in patients treated with an erythropoiesis-stimulating agent (ESA), to maintain adequate serum transferrin and ferritin levels.

The recommended dietary intake and supplements of vitamins in adult haemodialysis patients is presented in Table 8.2.

Chapter 8

Table 8.2 Recommended dietary intake and supplements of vitamins in adult haemodialysis patients (adopted from EBPG guideline on nutrition).

Vitamins	Daily recommendation
Thiamine (B$_1$)	1.1–1.2 mg supplement
Riboflavin (B$_2$)	1.1–1.3 mg supplement
Pyridoxine (B$_6$)	10 mg supplement
Ascorbic acid (C)	75–90 mg supplement
Folic acid	1 mg supplement
Cobalamin (B$_{12}$)	2.4 mg supplement
Niacin (B$_3$)	14–16 mg supplement
Biotin (B$_8$)	30 μg supplement
Pantothenic acid (B$_5$)	5 mg supplement
Retinol (A)	700–900 μg intake – no supplement
A-tocopherol (E)	400–800 IU supplement
Vitamin K	90–120 μg intake – no supplement

How does replacement therapy alter the dietary needs of patients with chronic kidney disease? Do the needs differ between peritoneal dialysis and haemodialysis?

Dietary recommendations for patients undergoing dialysis differ significantly from the recommendations for pre-end-stage CKD patients. The main difference is in protein intake. Both haemodialysis (HD) and peritoneal dialysis (PD) cause protein and amino acid losses during the dialysis. These losses can be as high as 10–12 g/session of HD and 4–12 g/day for PD patients, while in cases of peritonitis these losses can increase by up to 70%. Therefore, protein losses should be replaced for the achievement of a positive nitrogen balance in these patients. Dietary intake in stable haemodialysis patients should be at least 1.2 g/kg IBW/day, with emphasis being placed on proteins of high biological value (protein mainly from animal sources, such as meat, poultry, eggs, dairy products, fish and soy). Moving to PD patients, protein intake of 1.0 g/kg IBW/day is considered the minimum for stable, non-catabolic patients. Higher levels of protein intake are recommended for patients with peritonitis or catabolic stress, in which an intake of 1.5 g/kg IBW/day is suggested.

In addition to protein requirements, fluid restriction also differs in dialysis patients. In haemodialysis, when urine production diminishes, fluid intake should be limited to 500 ml/day + previous day's urine output. Anuric patients are advised to take 500–750 ml/day maximum in order to keep intradialytic weight gain to less than 2.5 kg over the weekend.

In PD patients, fluid allowance may be a bit more flexible owing to varying fluid removal by the PD bag prescription as a result of the dextrose concentrations of the dialysate. However, PD patients are advised to limit their fluid intake, as the excessive use of higher concentrate PD bags can result in undesirable weight gain and damage to the peritoneum.

Chapter 8

Finally, in HD patients, close monitoring of potassium is essential, as hyperkalaemia is common in this population. In PD patients, potassium is easily removed by the dialysate and usually there is no need for potassium restriction.

What are the main reasons contributing to anaemia in chronic kidney disease? How should anaemia be treated?

According to NKF KDOQI guidelines, anaemia in CKD is defined as haemoglobin less than 11 g/dl in pre-menopausal women and less than 12 g/dl in adult males and postmenopausal women. The main causes for anaemia in CKD are:

- reduced production of erythropoietin by the kidneys
- iron deficiency
- folate and B_{12} deficiency
- Lower red blood survival, caused mainly by uraemia

The management of anaemia in CKD includes the correction of iron deficiency, which is crucial before the initiation of treatment with ESAs. Iron supplementation is usually given orally in non-dialysed renal patients, while intravenous supplementation is preferred for HD patients. Adequate folate and B_{12} intakes, through diet and/or supplements, can assure the prevention of pernicious anaemia, while ESAs, such as epoetin alfa (Eprex), epoetin beta (NeoRecormon), darbepoetin alfa (Aranesp), should be offered to patients in the advanced stages of kidney disease, especially in those approaching dialysis.

What is intradialytic parenteral nutrition?

Intradialytic parenteral nutrition (IDPN) is the provision of nutrients intravenously through the venous drip chamber of a haemodialysis machine. According to NKF KDOQI, IDPN may be beneficial for malnourished patients or for those who are unable to meet their nutritional needs by oral nutrition. IDPN solutions usually provide amino acids and dextrose, while lipids can be added when there is a need for an increased energy intake. Vitamins and trace elements are not usually added in IDPN, as these additives can be lost in the dialysate. The use of IDPN in HD patients appears to be associated with decreased mortality and the improvement of prealbumin levels. However, the data supporting the use of IDPN are weak; therefore, a clear recommendation for its use cannot be made.

Table 8.3 Nutrition-related adverse effects of immunosuppressive therapy in transplanted patients.

Medication	Adverse effect
Corticosteroids	Glucose intolerance Weight gain Negative nitrogen balance Fluid retention Osteoporosis
Cyclosporine	Hyperkalaemia Hyperlipidaemia Weight gain
Mycophenolate mofetil	Gastrointestinal disturbances Hyperlipidaemia
Tacrolimus	Glucose intolerance Gastrointestinal disturbances

What are the dietary recommendations for patients with recent renal transplantation? How do they change in the long-term management of those patients?

After transplantation, provided that the graft is well functioning, most dietary restrictions imposed pre-dialysis and during the dialysis periods are not necessary. Although diet may be more liberal after transplantation, nutrition is an important part of the treatment of transplanted patients, mainly because of the metabolic effects of immunosuppressive therapy.

Immunosuppressive agents used for the prevention of graft rejection have adverse effects that could alter nutritional recommendations in transplanted patients (Table 8.3). Moreover, susceptibility to oral and throat infections due to immunosuppressants may limit the ability of eating, resulting in inadequate nutritional intake.

The first two months after transplantation, namely the acute post-transplant phase, a high-protein diet (1.2–1.3 g/kg IBW) is generally recommended to prevent a negative nitrogen balance, in combination with sufficient energy intake (30–35 kcal/kg IBW per day). In this phase strict sodium restriction is usually necessary (80–100 mmol/day/1000–2300 mg/day), as the dose of corticosteroids is rather high and there is a danger of fluid retention and hypertension. In the event of hyperkalaemia, potassium restrictions should be applied. As hypophosphataemia and hypomagnesaemia are common after transplantation, patients are encouraged to choose phosphate- and magnesium-rich foods (e.g. wholegrain products, nuts and seeds, low-fat dairy products, dried fruits), and in the event of abnormal serum values, supplemental intake may be chosen.

In the long term, an important problem that has to be solved is weight gain and the prevention of obesity. Advice on healthy eating should be given to patients in order to maintain a normal BMI. In cases of hyperlipidaemia due to the immunosuppressive therapy, dietary advice for lipid lowering should be applied. Regarding protein intake, it should be individualised, according to the graft function and the patient's needs. High-protein diets should be avoided, though, because of the danger of protein-induced hyperfiltration. A protein intake of 1.0 g/kg IBW is considered sufficient for the majority of stable transplanted patients, with good graft function.

In the event of graft rejection or its functional decline, recommendations should be adjusted according to the remnant renal function and the GFR of the graft.

Further reading

Beto JA, Bansal VK (2004) Medical nutrition therapy in chronic renal failure: Integrating clinical practice guidelines. *Journal of the American Dietetic Association* **104**: 404–9.

Block GA, Hulbert-Shearon TE, Levin NW, Port FK (1998) Association of serum phosphorus and calcium x phosphate product with mortality risk in chronic hemodialysis patients: A national study. *American Journal of Kidney Diseases* **31**(4): 607–17.

Byham-Gray L, Wiesen Karen (2004) *A Clinical Guide to Nutrition Care in Kidney Disease*. American Dietetic Association, Chicago.

Cano NJM, Fouques D, Roth H *et al.* (2007) French Study Group for Nutrition in Dialysis: Intradialytic parenteral nutrition does not improve survival in malnourished hemodialysis patients: A 2-year multi-center, prospective, randomized study. *Journal of the American Society of Nephrology* **18**: 2583–91.

Chazot C, Shahmir E, Matias B *et al.* (1997) Dialytic nutrition: Provision of amino acids in dialysate hemodialysis. *Kidney International* **52**(6): 1663–70.

Dieticians Special Interest Group (2002) *European Guidelines for the Nutritional Care of Adult Renal Patients*. European Dialysis and Transplantation Nurses Association/European Renal Care Association, http://www.eesc.europa.eu/self-and-coregulation/documents/codes/private/086-private-act.pdf, [accessed 18th February 2010].

Eyre S, Attman PO (2008) Protein restriction and body composition in renal disease. *Journal of Renal Nutrition* **18**: 167–86.

Foulks C J (1999) An evidence-based evaluation of intradialytic parenteral nutrition. *American Journal of Kidney Diseases* **33**(1): 186–92.

Fouque D (1996) Nephrotic syndrome and protein metabolism. *Nephrologie* **17**: 279–82.

Fouque D, Laville M, Boissel JP (2006) Low protein diets for chronic kidney disease in non diabetic adults. *Cochrane Database of Systematic Reviews 2006*, Issue 2. Art. No.: CD001892. DOI: 10.1002/14651858.CD001892.pub2. The Cochrane Library, 2006, issue 3.

Fouque D, Vennegoor M, ter Wee P *et al.* (2007) EBPG guideline on nutrition. *Nephrology Dialysis Transplantation* **22**(suppl. 2): S45–87.

Kaysen GA (1992) Nutritional management of nephritic syndrome. *Journal of Renal Nutrition* **2**: 50–8.

Kopple JD, Massry SG (2004) *Kopple and Massry's nutritional management of renal disease*, (2nd edn). Lippincott Williams & Wilkins, Philadelphia.

Levey AS, Greene T, Sarnak MJ *et al.* (2006) Effect of dietary protein restriction on the progression of kidney disease: Long-term follow-up of the Modification of Diet in Renal Disease (MDRD) Study. *American Journal of Kidney Diseases* **48**(6): 879–88.

Mansy H, Goodship TH, Tapson JS *et al.* (1989) Effect of a high protein diet in patients with the nephrotic syndrome. *Clinical Science (London)* **77**(4): 445–51.

Moe S, Drüeke T, Cunningham J *et al.* (2006) Definition, evaluation, and classification of renal osteodystrophy: A position statement from Kidney Disease: Improving Global Outcomes (KDIGO). *Kidney International* **69**: 1945–53.

National Kidney Foundation (2000) K/DOQI clinical practice guidelines for nutrition in CRF. *American Journal of Kidney Diseases* **35**(6, suppl. 2): S9, S56–63.

National Kidney Foundation (2005) K/DOQI clinical practice guidelines in cardiovascular disease in dialysis patients. *American Journal of Kidney Diseases* **45**(S3): 16–153.

National Kidney Foundation (2006) K/DOQI clinical practice guidelines and clinical practice recommendations for anemia in chronic kidney disease. *American Journal of Kidney Diseases* **47**(5, suppl. 3): S11–145.

Slatopolsky E (1998) The role of calcium, phosphorus and vitamin D metabolism in the development of secondary hyperparathyroidism. *Nephrology Dialysis Transplantation* **13**(suppl. 3): 3–8.

Thomas B (2007) *Manual of Dietetic Practice*, (3rd edn). Blackwell Science Ltd, Oxford.

Chapter 8

Chapter 9

Pulmonary Diseases

Charilaos Dimosthenopoulos, Meropi Kontogianni and Kalliopi-Anna Poulia

What is the respiratory quotient and is it important for patients with pulmonary diseases?

All macronutrients (i.e. proteins, carbohydrates and fats) are metabolised to carbon dioxide (CO_2) and water in the presence of oxygen. The ratio of CO_2 produced to oxygen consumed is referred to as the 'respiratory quotient' (RQ). Generally, the RQ of fat is 0.70, of protein 0.82, of carbohydrates 1.00, of ethanol 0.67 and of mixed fuels (i.e. carbohydrates, fat, protein and ethanol) 0.85. According to the RQ, a potential benefit may arise from increasing fat percentage in the pulmonary patient's diet; however, high levels of fat may not be well tolerated. Furthermore, excess calories are more significant in the production of CO_2 than the carbohydrate/fat ratio and fat may be preferred as an energy source for patients with severe dyspnoea, hypercapnia or the patient weaning from mechanical ventilation, since less CO_2 is produced compared to carbohydrate metabolism.

How does chronic obstructive pulmonary disease affect nutritional status?

Chronic obstructive pulmonary disease (COPD) is a progressively debilitating disease, which includes bronchitis and emphysema. In bronchitis, increased airway restriction is the result of increased bronchial secretions and bronchospasm. In emphysema, airway restriction is mainly the result of collapsible airways. The patient with bronchitis may be of optimal weight or even overweight, often with oedema and with frequent pulmonary infections, hypoxia and hypercapnia. Conversely, the patient with emphysema is usually thin, without oedema and relatively well oxygenated and usually exhibits moderately elevated blood CO_2 levels during the late stages of the disease. In these patients, weight loss significantly affects patient morbidity and mortality and is mainly attributed to increased energy expenditure (increased expenditure for respiration and because of frequent infections) and inadequate food intake.

What are the main dietary goals for patients with chronic obstructive pulmonary disease and their macronutrient needs?

The preservation of a normal weight (by providing small, frequent and energy-dense meals, high-energy oral supplements and restriction of aerophagia), the treatment of water imbalances and nutrient–drug interactions (especially due to corticosteroids, antibiotics and bronchodilators) are the main goals of nutritional management.

With regard to energy needs, these can be estimated using the Harris-Benedict equation (see Chapter 2) or with indirect calorimetry. In the presence of oedema, dry body weight should be estimated. In the case of infections and fever, energy needs may be increased; however, high intakes (e.g. >1.5 times resting energy expenditure) are not recommended since they may burden the respiratory system. Adequate amounts of protein (i.e. 1–1.5 g/kg dry body weight) are essential for optimal immune and pulmonary function. Moreover, for the achievement of a proper RQ, a balanced macronutrient intake (e.g. 15–20% of daily energy intake from protein, 40–55% from carbohydrates and 30–45% from fat) is crucial.

What is cystic fibrosis and what are its main nutritional implications?

Cystic fibrosis (CF) is an inherited disorder which leads to significant dysfunction of the exocrine glands and results in chronic lung disease, pancreatic insufficiency with subsequent malabsorption and high concentrations of sodium and chloride in sweat. Deterioration of pulmonary function may increase nutrient requirements somewhat, but probably affects nutrition more by adversely affecting intake, particularly during acute exacerbations and in older children with severe pulmonary disease. Pancreatic insufficiency severely limits the absorption of fat, a major energy source of most diets. Thus, the cause of malnutrition in infants and children with this disease can be both primary (i.e. inadequate nutrient intake) and secondary (i.e. faecal loss of protein and, particularly, of fat). The latter cause usually can be controlled with appropriate pancreatic enzyme replacement because there does not seem to be a primary defect in energy metabolism associated with the disease. Regarding nutritional management goals, the restriction of malabsorption by optimal pancreatic enzyme replacement therapy and proper diet, as well as the coverage of energy and nutrient needs, are the cornerstones of diet therapy.

How can energy needs for patients with cystic fibrosis be assessed?

Traditionally, a high-energy, high-protein, low-fat diet has been advocated for patients with CF, although in many patients with advanced disease intakes of both protein and energy, but especially energy, are far lower than recommended. The energy needs of patients with CF depend on the degree of pulmonary disease, physical activity and the degree of malabsorption. CF patients have higher energy needs (120–150% of the recommended daily intake) for age and sex. Energy requirements vary a lot and depend on factors such as basic metabolic rate, sex, age, level of physical activity and presence of possible respiratory infection. The energy needs of CF patients can be assessed by indirect calorimetry, which in this case is a relatively difficult process. For the estimation of energy needs of patients with CF it is necessary to estimate the basal metabolic rate (BMR) using the existing equations. The daily energy requirements can be estimated by multiplying BMR by the physical activity factor and adding the disease factor (0.0–0.5), which is related to the degree of pulmonary function and the percentage of the exhaled air in 1 second (forced expiratory volume: FEV_1).

What are the macro- and micronutrient requirements for patients with cystic fibrosis?

Patients with CF have higher protein requirements [120% of the recommended nutrient intake (RNI) owing to increased losses] and relatively high fat requirements (35–40%), despite malabsorption, in order to provide adequate energy. A beneficial effect of docosahexaenoic acid on CF pathology has been suggested by recent studies, but this suggestion requires further critical evaluation. The content of fibre in the diet depends on the possible presence of constipation. As far as concerns micronutrients, CF patients are more likely to present with fat-soluble vitamin (A, D, E or even K) deficiency, rather than water-soluble vitamin deficiency (C and B complex). Sodium, zinc and iron may have to be supplemented in the diet of CF patients.

What dietary factors can play a favourable role in the management of patients with asthma?

Several studies have examined the possible role of nutrients and food groups on asthma patients. Evidence suggests that the suboptimum intake of antioxidants could increase the risk of asthma. Recent publications support the favourable effect of the adherence to the Mediterranean diet and to increased fruit intake, wholegrain cereals and flavonoid-rich foods in asthma prevention and treatment, while adherence to the Mediterranean diet during pregnancy lowers the risk of the development of asthma and atopy in the neonate and during its childhood. Especially in children, a high fruit intake and adherence to the Mediterranean diet has been associated with the improvement of the symptoms of asthma and rhinitis, while it has been shown to be an independent protective factor for wheezing, irrespective of obesity and physical activity. Moreover, increased magnesium, selenium, zinc and copper intake and the limitation in sodium intake have also been shown to have a favourable effect. In epidemiological studies, in populations with increased

Chapter 9

omega-3 fatty acids intake (i.e. Eskimos), a lower prevalence of asthma has been reported. The possible mechanism of the protective effect of omega-3 fatty acids probably rests with their anti-inflammatory properties, but this positive effect has not been confirmed in clinical studies. Apart from the role of nutrients, the achievement and maintenance of a healthy body weight and an overall nutritional balance have been shown to improve respiratory function in obese patients.

Do nutritional needs alter in patients with pneumonia?

Patients with pneumonia usually have increased energy needs because of the elevated body temperature that is observed in them. These patients should be advised to increase their energy intake of nutrient-dense foods and increase their vitamin and mineral intake. Moreover, these patients often have increased fluid needs owing to increased fluid loss caused by sweating and/or diarrhoea. Therefore, the sufficient provision of liquids is essential.

Further reading

Barros, R, Moreira A, Fonseca J et al. (2008) Adherence to the Mediterranean diet and fresh fruit intake are associated with improved asthma control. *Allergy* **63**: 917–23.

Castro-Rodriguez JA, Garcia-Marcos L, Alfonseda Rojas JD et al. (2008) Mediterranean diet as a protective factor for wheezing in preschool children. *Journal of Pediatrics* **152**: 823–8.

Eneli IU, Skybo T, Camargo CA Jr (2008) Weight loss and asthma: A systematic review. *Thorax* **63**: 671–6.

Gao J, Gao X, Li W et al. (2008) Observational studies on the effect of dietary antioxidants on asthma: A meta-analysis. *Respirology* **13**: 528–36.

Ramsey BW, Farrell PM, Pencharz P (1992) Nutritional assessment and management in cystic fibrosis: A consensus report. The Consensus Committee. *American Journal of Clinical Nutrition* **55**(1): 108–16.

Schols AMWJ (2000) Nutrition in chronic obstructive pulmonary disease. *Current Opinion in Pulmonary Medicine* **6**: 110–15.

Stallings VA, Stark LJ, Robinson KA et al. (2008) Evidence-based practice recommendations for nutrition-related management of children and adults with cystic fibrosis and pancreatic insufficiency: Results of a systematic review. *Journal of the American Dietetic Association* **108**(5): 832–9.

Thomas B (2007) *Manual of Dietetic Practice*, (3rd edn). Blackwell Science Ltd, Oxford.

Van Biervliet S, Vande Velde S, Van Biervliet JP, Robberecht E. (2008) The effect of zinc supplements in cystic fibrosis patients. *Annals of Nutrition & Metabolism* **52**(2): 152–6.

Winklhofer-Roob BM (2000) Cystic fibrosis: Nutritional status and micronutrients. *Current Opinion in Clinical Nutrition and Metabolic Care* **3**(4): 293–7.

Chapter 10

Life Expectancy

Evangelia Manglara

Introduction

The rise in life expectancy (which is 75 years for men and 80 years for women today) is mainly due to better sanitation, hygiene and health care, reduced infant mortality and the use of antibiotics and vaccines. Lifespan may also be increased by the therapeutic use of calorie restriction, which seems to improve health as well.

What are the main data on experimental animals indicating that calorie restriction prolongs life expectancy?

In 1935, it was first reported that calorie restriction extended lifespan in rats. Subsequent data have shown that calorie intake reduction without malnutrition slows ageing and prolongs maximum lifespan in other species as well. Maximum lifespan in rodents is also prolonged by intermittent fasting.

What are the main possible mechanisms involved?

The five main possible mechanisms are:

- reduced production of reactive oxygen species
- decreased circulating T_3 levels and sympathetic nervous system activity
- decreased plasma inflammatory cytokine concentrations
- protection against ageing-associated immune function deterioration
- increased expression of protein chaperones and neurotrophic factors.

Does energy restriction have the same effect on humans?

Although there are no validated biomarkers of ageing and it is impracticable to conduct randomised, diet-controlled, long-term survival studies in humans, epidemiologic data show that energy restriction may positively affect factors involved in the pathogenesis of ageing and life expectancy in humans. Coronary heart disease mortality rates, which had declined during World War II food shortages in Europe, rose again after the end of the war. In addition, Okinawa inhabitants, who ate fewer calories than Japanese, had lower cardiovascular disease and cancer rates. The causal association between energy restriction and longevity, however, has not been definitely proven.

What are the changes in different biomarkers observed with calorie restriction in humans?

There are several changes:

- low percentage of body fat
- low systolic and diastolic blood pressures
- markedly improved lipid profile
- increased insulin sensitivity
- low plasma concentrations of inflammatory markers
- low levels of circulating growth factors
- low serum concentrations of T_3.

Moreover, left ventricular diastolic function in calorie-restricted persons was similar to that of persons 16 years younger.

What happens with calorie restriction in obese patients?

Calorie restriction leading to weight loss improves numerous obesity-associated risk factors. Recent studies have also shown that long-term weight loss caused by bariatric-surgery-induced calorie restriction reduces mortality in extremely obese individuals.

What is the optimal calorie intake to prolong life?

The optimal calorie intake for life prolongation is not known. However, the available data suggest that calorie restriction with adequate nutrient intake in humans is as beneficial as in animal models. It can increase life expectancy and enhance late-life quality by lessening chronic disease burden. It must be noted, though, that energy restriction may be harmful for certain populations, such as lean individuals with extremely low body fat stores.

Chapter 10

What is the effect of the genetic factor?

Some people are genetically predisposed to live longer. Studies show that familial longevity is inherited, the mortality of centenarian siblings is almost half throughout life and their relative risk to reach 100 is higher than in the general population. Centenarian offspring also show lower risk of mortality and most centenarians have intact cognitive function even after the age of 90.

Does diet type influence survival?

Certainly, there are clear indications of that. A large population-based prospective investigation conducted on 22,043 adults in Greece showed an inverse association with greater adherence to the Mediterranean diet for both death due to coronary heart disease and death from cancer.

In addition, another study conducted in China showed that a fruit-rich diet was related to lower mortality, while a diet rich in meat was associated with higher diabetes risk and a slightly higher risk of total mortality.

In accordance with the above results are the data of an Italian study showing that in older subjects the 'olive oil and salad' dietary pattern (which included the high intake of olive oil, raw vegetables, soups and poultry) was inversely associated with overall mortality, whereas the 'pasta and meat' pattern (including pasta, tomato sauce, red meat, processed meat, animal fat, white bread and wine) was associated with increased overall mortality.

It is also worth noting that the Greek study mentioned above showed that adherence to a Mediterranean diet was essentially unrelated to body mass index (BMI), with small variations depending on model choice and with no practical consequences.

A recent report from Finland clearly showed that the long-term change in population diets (mainly a reduction of saturated fat and an increase of unsaturated fat intake) resulted in a major increase in life expectancy and in an 80% reduction in annual cardiovascular disease mortality rates.

It was mentioned above that the Mediterranean diet is associated with an increased life expectancy in the general population. What has been shown in patients with coronary heart disease?

The association between the degree of adherence to the Mediterranean diet and survival of patients with diagnosed coronary heart disease (CHD) at enrolment was examined in a population-based prospective study of 1302 Greek men and women. The results showed that a greater adherence to the Mediterranean diet was associated with a significantly lower mortality rate among patients with prevalent CHD at enrolment.

In addition, similar results were shown in a French study, the so-called Lyon Diet Heart Study, a randomised secondary prevention trial designed to test whether a Mediterranean diet may lower recurrence rates after a first

Chapter 10

myocardial infarction. The conclusion was that the cardioprotective effect of the Mediterranean diet pattern was maintained up to four years after the initial infarction. The relationships of recurrence to major traditional risk factors, such as high blood cholesterol and blood pressure, were qualitatively unaltered. Therefore, further trials are needed.

How could one summarise the above data?

There are indirect indications that:

- calorie restriction in adults may prolong lifespan
- a greater adherence to the Mediterranean type of diet is associated with increased survival.

Further reading

Cai H, Shu XO, Gao YT et al. (2007) A prospective study of dietary patterns and mortality in Chinese women. *Epidemiology* **18**(3): 393–401.

Fontana L, Klein S (2007) Aging, adiposity, and calorie restriction. *Journal of the American Medical Association* **297**(9): 986–94.

Hunter P (2007) Is eternal youth scientifically plausible? *EMBO Reports* **8**(1): 18–20.

de Lorgeril M, Salen P, Martin JL et al. (1999) Mediterranean diet, traditional risk factors, and the rate of cardiovascular complications after myocardial infarction: Final report of the Lyon Diet Heart Study. *Circulation* **99**(6): 733–5.

Masala G, Ceroti M, Pala V et al. (2007) A dietary pattern rich in olive oil and raw vegetables is associated with lower mortality in Italian elderly subjects. *British Journal of Nutrition* **98**(2): 406–15.

Puca AA, Chatgilialoglu C, Ferreri C et al. (2007) Lipid metabolism and diet: Possible mechanisms of slow aging. *International Journal of Biochemistry and Cell Biology* **40**(3): 324–33.

Pusca P (2009) Fat and heart disease: Yes we can make a change: The case of North Karelia (Finland). *Annals of Nutrition & Metabolism* **54**(suppl. 1): 33–8.

Trichopoulou A, Bamia C, Trichopoulos D (2005) Mediterranean diet and survival among patients with coronary heart disease in Greece. *Archives of Internal Medicine* **165**: 929–35.

Trichopoulou A, Costacou T, Bamia C, Trichopoulos D (2003) Adherence to a Mediterranean diet and survival in a Greek population. *New England Journal of Medicine* **348**(26): 2599–608.

Trichopoulou A, Naska A, Orfanos P, Trichopoulos D (2005) Mediterranean diet in relation to body mass index and waist-to-hip ratio: The Greek European Prospective Investigation into Cancer and Nutrition Study. *American Journal of Clinical Nutrition* **82**: 935–40.

Trichopoulou A, Psaltopoulou T, Orfanos P et al. (2007) Low-carbohydrate-high-protein diet and long-term survival in a general population cohort. *European Journal of Clinical Nutrition* **61**: 575–81.

Chapter 10

Chapter 11
HIV/AIDS

Kalliopi-Anna Poulia

What is HIV/AIDS disease and what are the main modes of transmission?

Acquired immunodeficiency syndrome (AIDS) is a disorder resulting from the infection with the human immunodeficiency virus (HIV), which leads to a profound immunosuppression and high susceptibility to life-threatening opportunistic infections and malignancies. It was first reported in 1981.

HIV infection can be transmitted by:

- unprotected vaginal and anal sexual intercourse
- receipt of infected blood and blood products (sharing injecting equipment between drug users, occupational accidents with needle stick injuries, infusion of contaminated blood products)
- from the infected mother to the child during pregnancy, birth or breast-feeding (vertical transmission).

How is HIV disease classified?

According to the Centers of Disease Control (CDC) in the USA, HIV disease is classified in nine categories according to the symptoms and the CD4 cell count, as described in Table 11.1.

What are the main goals of nutritional care for HIV-positive patients?

Since malnutrition is one of the most common problems in patients with HIV/AIDS, nutritional care aims predominately at the efficient provision of nutrients and the maintenance of body weight and lean body mass within normal levels. Moreover, the delay of wasting syndrome and the early detection and treatment of the metabolic disturbances due to the disease or

Table 11.1 Classification of HIV disease according to the Centers of Disease Control in the USA.

CD4 lymphocytes count	Symptoms			
	A Asymptomatic disease, acute retroviral syndrome, generalised lymphadenopathy	B Symptoms of AIDS-related complex	C AIDS-defining conditions
>500/μL	A1		B1	C1
200–499/μL	A2		B2	C2
<200/μL	A3		B3	C3

All patients in categories C1, B2, C2, A3, B3 and C3 are characterised as patients with AIDS.

the antiretroviral therapy are of main concern. Finally, patients with HIV/AIDS should be provided with nutritional advice tailored to their specific needs, the possible side effects of their medications and their lifestyles.

What are the main factors precipitating weight loss and wasting in HIV disease?

The most common nutritional problem in symptomatic HIV disease is weight loss or wasting. Although its severity and frequency appear to be reduced by the use of antiretroviral therapy, it remains a problem. Since malnutrition can reduce the quality of life and increase morbidity and mortality in these patients, the early detection and treatment of the underlying cause of insufficient nutrient intake is of vital importance.

Malnutrition in HIV patients can often be attributed to:

- reduced food intake, due to psychological an neurological problems, sore mouth or side effects of their medication (i.e. anorexia, vomiting, nausea)
- altered metabolic needs due to the progression of the disease
- malabsorption, especially in patients with chronic diarrhoea caused by gastrointestinal pathogens, by medication or by the HIV disease itself.

What are the nutritional needs of an asymptomatic or weight stable patient with HIV infection?

The main goal for asymptomatic or weight stable HIV-positive patients is to optimise food intake and to ensure the adequate intake of nutrients. Unintentional weight loss should be avoided by the sufficient provision of energy and protein. Although the micronutrient requirements of HIV-positive patients are unknown, a multivitamin and mineral supplement, providing no more than 100% of dietary reference intake (DRI) or reference nutrient intake (RNI) could be prescribed in order to avoid deficiencies, especially when food intake is compromised.

What are the goals of the nutritional management of symptomatic patients with HIV infection?

The main goals of the nutritional management of symptomatic patients with HIV infection are:

- the preservation or increase of lean body mass
- adequate provision of macro- and micronutrients
- achievement and/or maintenance of a body weight within the normal values for body mass index (BMI)
- provision of symptomatic relief, according to the patient's needs.

How are the energy and protein needs in symptomatic HIV-positive patients calculated?

In being a part of the medical care team responsible for the management of HIV-positive patients, the clinical dietitian should have the ability to combine the available data from the nutritional assessment, the medical treatment and the patient's individual needs in order to provide tailor-made advice to the patient.

The energy needs of these patients vary greatly, according to the state of the disease, the presence of problems that could compromise absorption and the utilisation of nutrients. Ideally, energy needs should be calculated by indirect calorimetry. However, in the clinical setting, energy needs could be calculated, with limited accuracy though, by the use of equations such as the Harris-Benedict or Schofield equations, taking into account the relative stress factors according to the overall health status of the patient. Energy requirements are likely to increase by 10% to maintain body weight and physical activity in asymptomatic HIV-infected adults. During symptomatic HIV, and subsequently during AIDS, energy requirements increase by approximately 20–30% to maintain adult body weight.

Protein needs in HIV-positive patients are considered relatively high. A dietary protein intake of 1.5–2 g/kg is considered adequate for the majority of patients. Likewise, providing 20% of a patient's daily energy intake as protein seems to cover the needs of HIV-infected patients, given the fact that their energy needs are high. These recommendations may differentiate in patients with kidney or hepatic disease. In these cases, the relevant recommendations for non-HIV patients should be followed.

Do vitamin and mineral needs differ in symptomatic HIV-positive patients?

The exact micronutrient needs of HIV-positive patients are not established yet. According to the available data, HIV-positive patients seem to have lower levels of vitamin A, B_6, C and E in the bloodstream. These data possibly suggest that HIV-positive patients may need these vitamins more than the healthy population does.

What is highly active antiretroviral therapy?

'Highly active antiretroviral therapy' (HAART) is a term used to describe the use of a combination of antiretroviral drugs for the treatment of HIV infection. The main antiretroviral drugs that are used for HIV-positive subjects are categorised according to the phase of the retrovirus life cycle that the drugs inhibit, as follows:

- nucleoside and non-nucleoside reverse transcriptase inhibitors (NRTIs and nNRTIs respectively) inhibit reverse transcription of the virus.
- protease inhibitors (PIs) inhibit the activity of protease (an enzyme used by HIV to cleave nascent proteins for the final assembly of new virons).
- integrase inhibitors inhibit integrase, the enzyme that is responsible for the integration of viral DNA into the DNA of the host cell.
- fusion inhibitors interfere with the binding, fusion and entry of the HIV virus to the host cell.
- maturation inhibitors inhibit the last step of virus production, by blocking the formation of the capsid protein of the virus.

What are the main nutrition-related side effects of highly active antiretroviral therapy?

The use of HAART has transformed HIV infection from an acute illness to a manageable chronic condition. However, the significant decrease in mortality of HIV patients and the increase in their life expectancy have been accompanied by several clinical and metabolic complications. Nutrition-related side effects have been shown to correlate negatively with quality-of-life measures in people infected with HIV. The most common gastrointestinal adverse effects include nausea, vomiting, dyspepsia, anorexia, abdominal pain, chewing/swallowing difficulties and taste alterations. Usually, these effects lose their intensity after the first month of treatment. If they persist, they may compromise dietary intake, and a change in the drug regimen should be considered. Providing specific strategies to support patients through these challenges is an important part of nutritional therapy.

The main metabolic complication is described as 'HAART-induced lipodystrophy syndrome', which includes:

- lipoatrophy (face, extremities and buttocks)
- fat accumulation (abdomen, dorsocervical or supraclavicular fat pad – buffalo hump)
- dyslipidaemia [hypertriglyceridaemia, hypercholesterolaemia and low high-density lipoprotein (HDL) cholesterol]
- insulin resistance and glucose intolerance
- lactic acidosis.

What is the role of nutrition in the management of HAART-induced dyslipidaemia?

In the absence of results from randomised, controlled clinical trials evaluating specific dietary interventions in HIV-infected patients with lipid disorders, the current recommendations for the management of dyslipidaemia in HIV-infected patients receiving HAART do not differ from the recommendations for the non-HIV-infected population. It is suggested that HIV-infected patients with dyslipidaemia should follow the National Cholesterol Education Program Adult Treatment Panel III (NCEP ATP III) recommendations, which include dietary restriction of total fat to 25–35% of total energy intake, saturated fat to less than 7% of total calories, dietary cholesterol to less than 200 mg per day, use of plant sterols (2 g/d) and attainment of a prudent diet increased with a high intake of dietary fibre (10–25 g/d). Recent data also support the use of a Mediterranean diet pattern (low in saturated fat, without a severe restriction of monounsaturated or omega-3 polyunsaturated fat, replacing some of the complex carbohydrates with monounsaturated fatty acids). Increased physical activity or exercise, especially weight-bearing exercise in combination with aerobic activities, could benefit patients, by reserving muscle mass and improving cardiovascular health. Lifestyle changes recommended for the treatment of isolated hypertriglyceridaemia, in addition to reduced fat intake and exercise, include reduction in alcohol and refined-sugars intake.

What is AIDS wasting syndrome and how can it be managed?

'Wasting syndrome' is a term used to describe unintentional weight loss (>10% of the usual body weight) in combination with diarrhoea, fatigue and/or fever for a period of more than 30 days. The weight loss concerns mainly the loss of lean body mass and, secondarily, fat mass. Wasting can contribute to the deterioration of a patient's immune system and is connected with high rates of mortality and usually signals that the HIV-infection is progressing to AIDS.

Detailed dietary assessment should be performed regularly in HIV-infected patients to ensure the early detection of wasting syndrome. When and if it is identified, certain actions should take place in order to maximise dietary intake of the patient and halt their weight loss. Dietary advice should focus on energy- and nutrient-dense foods, while meal planning should be the first priority for these patients. Food enrichment and food fortification could also improve the nutrient intake. If the patient's dietary intake remains compromised, oral supplements could be used.

If the patient fails to attain a sufficient dietary intake, the use of artificial nutrition should be considered. Enteral and parenteral nutrition could be used in order to preserve the patient's nutritional status.

Does omega-3 fatty acid intake benefit patients with HIV infection?

Omega-3 fatty acids – namely eicosapentaenoic and docosahexaenoic acid – have been shown to be effective for lowering triglycerides in patients with

HIV-associated dyslipidaemia. A 16-week randomised study in patients with HAART-associated hypertriglyceridaemia showed that fish oil supplementation reduced plasma triglyceride by 20%. Other studies have demonstrated the benefits of omega-3 fatty acids as well. Omega-3 fatty acids may also have secondary benefits in decreasing bone resorption and decreasing markers of systemic inflammation.

What are the main strategies for reducing the danger of food- and water-borne illnesses?

HIV-infected patients, owing to their compromised immune system, are usually more vulnerable to food-borne illness than the non-infected population. Special care should be taken for the education of HIV-infected patients in the safe handling of food in order to minimise the danger of a food-borne illness. Strict hygiene measures should be taken during food preparation, and foods easily spoilt or of a high microbial load should be avoided (raw or semi-raw meat and fish, raw eggs, non-pasteurised milk and milk products, soft cheese and cheese with moulds, i.e. Roquefort or blue cheese). Moreover, attention should be paid to the expiry dates of food products and to the careful storing of food.

In the developed world, tap water is usually safe. If water comes from wells or rivers, it should be boiled before it is consumed. Ice cubes and cold drinks should also be prepared from safe water in order to avoid water-borne illnesses.

Further reading

ADA Reports (2004) Position of Dietitians of Canada and the American Dietetic Association: Nutrition intervention in the care of persons with human immunodeficiency virus infection. *Journal of the American Dietetic Association* **104**(9): 1425–41.

AHA Report (2001) Executive summary of the third report of the National Cholesterol Educational Program expert panel on detection, evaluation and treatment of high blood cholesterol in adults (Adult Treatment Panel III). *Journal of the American Medical Association* **285**: 2486–97.

Centers for Disease Control and Prevention (1992) 1993 Revised classification system for HIV infection and expanded surveillance case definition for AIDS among adolescents and adults. *Morbidity and Mortality Weekly Report* **41**: RR–17.

Dubé MP, Stein JH, Aberg JA *et al.* (2003) Guidelines for the evaluation and management of dyslipidemia in human immunodeficiency virus (HIV)-infected adults receiving antiretroviral therapy: Recommendations of the HIV Medical Association of the Infectious Disease Society of America and the Adult AIDS Clinical Trials Group. *Clinical Infectious Diseases* **37**(September): 613–27.

Chapter 11

Hadigan C (2003) Dietary habits and their association with metabolic abnormalities in human immunodeficiency virus-related lipodystrophy. *Clinical Infectious Diseases* **37**(suppl. 2): S101–4.

Joy T, Keogh HM, Hadigan C *et al.* (2007) Dietary fat intake and relationship to serum lipid levels in HIV-infected patients with metabolic abnormalities in the HAART era. *AIDS* **21**(12): 1591–600.

Leow MKS, Addy CL, Matzoros CS (2003) Human immunodeficiency virus/highly active antiretroviral therapy-associated metabolic syndrome: Clinical presentation, pathophysiology, and therapeutic strategies. *Journal of Clinical Endocrinology and Metabolism* **88**(5): 1961–76.

Leyes P, Martínez E, Forga Mde T (2008) Use of diet, nutritional supplements and exercise in HIV-infected patients receiving combination antiretroviral therapies: A systematic review. *Antiretroviral Therapy* **13**(2): 149–59.

Mangili A, Murman DH, Zampini AM, Wanke CA (2006) Nutrition and HIV infection: Review of weight loss and wasting in the era of highly active antiretroviral therapy from the Nutrition for Healthy Living cohort. *Clinical Infectious Diseases* **42**(6): 836–42.

Metroka CE, Truong P, Gotto AM Jr (2007) Treatment of HIV-associated dyslipidemia: A role for omega-3 fatty acids. *AIDS Reader* **17**(7): 362–73.

Ohm J, Hegele RA (2007) HIV-associated dyslipidaemia: Pathogenesis and treatment. *Lancet Infectious Diseases* **7**(12): 787–96.

Thomas B (2007) *Manual of Dietetic Practice*, (3rd edn). Blackwell Science Ltd, Oxford.

World Health Organization (2003) Nutrient Requirements for People Living with HIV/AIDS: Report of a technical consultation. WHO, Geneva.

Chapter 12

Metabolic Stress

Charilaos Dimosthenopoulos

Introduction

There are many conditions of metabolic stress, but the most important that require specific nutritional support are head injury, burns, surgery and systemic inflammatory response syndrome/multiple organ dysfunction syndrome.

How can a head injury patient be fed in order to meet their energy and protein requirements?

Head injury is a trauma of the head, with or without injury to the brain. Head injury is a condition that increases the metabolic responses and the nutritional needs of the whole body. The initial systemic response after injury is the condition of hypermetabolism and hypercatabolism. In the acute phase, head injury decreases the immunological and gastrointestinal functions, leads to hyperglycaemia and increases ventricular fluid and the levels of serum cytokines. The provision of an adequate supply of nutrients is associated with an improved patient outcome. Early and adequate nutrition, whether enteral or parenteral, is believed to be essential for the patient's health and for improving the outcome of their injury. The best route of nutritional administration (parenterally or enterally) and the best timing of administration (e.g. early versus late) should be established. Most of the related studies propose early feeding in order to achieve better outcomes related to the patient's survival and disability. A significant benefit of glutamine supplementation on the safety and efficacy of the treatment, decreased mortality, duration of stay and infectious morbidity in critical illness has been demonstrated by recent data of head-injured patients.

What methods of nutritional support are preferred in the case of head injury?

As mentioned above, head injury increases the body's metabolic responses and its nutritional demands and therefore the provision of an adequate supply of nutrients is associated with improved treatment outcomes. The two different routes for the administration of nutrition are total parenteral nutrition (TPN) or enteral nutrition (EN).

- **TPN** is used in severely head-injured patients, when there is no gastric function or after an extended period, when a patient is nil by mouth. There are studies that propose this mode of feeding in order to achieve a better treatment outcome following head injury.
- **EN** is preferred when there is gastric function, because of the lower risk of hyperglycaemia, infection and total cost. The route of administration can be through a percutaneous gastrostomy or jejunostomy tube or through percutaneous gastrojejunostomy. Recent studies suggest that an enteral formula containing glutamine and probiotics may decrease the infection rate and shorten the patient's stay in the intensive care unit. The presence of increased intracranial pressure and the position and the severity of the brain injury may determine the beginning of EN.

Most of the current studies have proved that when either parenteral or enteral feeding covers energy expenditure and nitrogen excretion, through equivalent quantities of feeding, almost the same outcome in the patient's treatment is achieved.

What are the classifications of burns?

When the skin is exposed to excessive heat (from fire), electricity or corrosive chemicals, the resulting tissue damage is known as a 'burn'. The estimation of the severity of burn is based on its depth and the percentage body surface that is burnt. Burns are generally categorised according to the severity of tissue damage, as follows:

- **First-degree burns:** They affect only the outer layer of the skin (epidermis) (e.g. mild sunburn). They are characterised by pain and redness and will heal within 5–10 days.
- **Second-degree burns:** They affect both the epidermis and the layer below it (the dermis). They are characterised by pain, redness and blisters and will heal in 10–14 days (for milder burns) or 25–35 days (when the depth of burn is greater). They require hospitalisation.
- **Third-degree burns:** They destroy the epidermis and dermis, and can involve all layers of the skin and subcutaneous fat, and even underlying bones, muscles and tendons. They are characterised by a white burn site, lack of sensation due to the destruction of the nerve endings, disturbed temperature control and a higher danger of infections. They require immediate hospitalisation.

What are the basic treatment goals for the nutritional care of the burn patient?

Severe burn patients present an extreme state of physiological stress and an overwhelming systemic metabolic response. They require specialised nutritional support, which is an integral part of multidisciplinary management. The main nutritional goals in the treatment of the burn patient are:

- Monitor nutritional status and provide specialised immune-enhancing nutrition.
- Estimate energy requirements and provide adequate calories to prevent weight loss of greater than 10% usual body weight.
- Provide adequate protein for positive nitrogen balance and maintenance or repletion of circulating proteins. The goal of nutritional therapy is to prevent rather than treat already established malnutrition, but protein degradation in burn patients proceeds despite adequate protein supplementation.
- Provide vitamin and mineral supplementation as indicated.
- Take into account the hormonal and metabolic changes resulting from a burn injury.

What is the role of protein in the treatment of burns?

Protein requirements are also increased in burn patients because of the increased catabolism of skeletal muscle, leading to average losses of 260 mg protein/kg/hr. Protein intake should vary between 1.5–2.0 g/kg of ideal body weight on a daily basis. Nitrogen balance should be assessed on a daily or weekly basis, using the Waxman equation. The rate of protein breakdown into amino acids and the reincorporation of these amino acids are important for collagen synthesis in wound healing as well as for the maintenance of visceral proteins for optimal organ function, especially the immune system. Maintenance of diaphragm and intercostal muscle mass is also important for survival to avoid the reduction of vital capacity and respiratory efficiency. In addition to the urinary losses from the degradation of muscle mass, nitrogen is lost from wound exudate, excision of burns and blood loss during surgery, leading to an extraordinarily negative nitrogen balance.

How are the nutrient needs of a burn patient calculated?

Burn injury increases the body's metabolic demands, and therefore nutritional requirements. Provision of an adequate supply of nutrients is believed to lower the incidence of metabolic abnormalities, thus reducing septic morbidity, and improving survival rates. The purpose of the nutritional assessment is to characterise the patient's nutritional status and recognise pre-existing malnutrition. This is essential for developing an appropriate nutritional regimen to treat specific nutritional disorders (e.g. thiamin replacement for alcoholic patients), to provide optimal repletion during the metabolic insult of the burn and multiple surgeries, to reduce morbidity and mortality, and to minimise any loss of muscle strength. Nutritional status is assessed in most patients by a variety of methods, such as anthropometric measurement, biochemical data, clinical signs and diet history (see Chapter 2). The traditional parameters of anthropometric, biochemical and clinical data will not be accurate in burn patients because the results are distorted by fluid resuscitation, surgeries and systemic inflammatory responses. For example, body weight, mid-arm circumference, blood count and visceral protein status are affected by fluid resuscitation and transfusion, and nitrogen balance is affected by burn exudate and immobility. Therefore, diet history becomes more important to nutritional assessments than usual.

Do certain vitamins contribute to the treatment of burns?

Critically ill burn patients present an increased free radical production, which is proportional to the severity of the burn, while micronutrient deficiencies are frequent after major burns. Burn patients have a high risk of negative trace element balances, which contribute to the imbalance in endogenous antioxidant capacity and the extension of primary lesions. As far as concerns the route of administration, the intravenous route has been proposed as more efficient than the enteral. The clinical evidence shows that several factors may determine the efficacy of antioxidant supplementation in burn patients. In severe burns, high doses of vitamin C contribute to a reduction of resuscitation fluid requirements by endothelial antioxidant mechanisms and should be administered to the burn patient in quantities equal to 5–10% of the recommended daily allowance (RDA). B-complex vitamins should be administered in quantities equal to 2–3 times of the RDA, vitamins A and D in quantities equal to twice the RDA and vitamins B_{12} and K once a week.

How are the fluid and electrolyte needs of a burn patient estimated?

It is of primary importance in the care and treatment of burn patients to monitor the electrolyte–fluid balance and to contribute to an accurate fluid resuscitation. Lactated Ringer's solution without dextrose is the fluid of choice, except in children under two, who should receive 5% dextrose in lactated Ringer's solution. The initial rate can be estimated by multiplying the estimated total body surface area (TBSA) burnt, using the appropriate graphs, by the weight in kilograms, which is divided by 4. The various formulas used for the estimation of the total volume of fluids needed in the first 24 hours are shown in Table 12.1.

The restoration of sodium losses in burn patients is essential, as mild or severe hyponatraemia (<135 mEq/l) can be present, mainly owing to extracellular sodium depletion, which follows all the changes that occur in cellular permeability. Hyperkalaemia is another characteristic of massive tissue necrosis.

Table 12.1 Resuscitation formulas.

Formula	Crystalloid volume	Colloid volume	Free water
Parkland	4 ml/kg/% TBSA burnt	None	None
Brooke	1.5 ml/kg/% TBSA burnt	0.5 ml/kg/% TBSA burnt	2.0 l
Galveston (paediatric)	5000 ml/m² TBSA burnt + 1500 ml/m²	None	None

TBSA = total body surface area.

What increases the risk of developing pressure sores?

Pressure sores are primarily developed by unrelieved pressure. There are numerous risk factors responsible for the development of pressure sores, which can be categorised as extrinsic or intrinsic. Sustained pressure, shearing forces, friction and moisture, mechanical loads on the skin and the soft tissues and body weight, age, sex, limitation in activity, dehydration and bowel and bladder incontinence, anaemia, poor nutritional status, medication and infection are some the most important risk factors involved in the aetiology and development of pressure sores.

What nutrients can contribute to the treatment of pressure sores?

Pressure ulcers are areas of damage to the skin and underlying tissue that usually occur over bony protrusions such as elbows, heels and hips. Pressure ulcers are caused most frequently by pressure, shear and friction. While unrelieved pressure, shearing forces and friction account for the mechanical aetiology of pressure ulcers, many other conditions can also predispose an individual to pressure ulcers. Pressure sores and malnutrition usually coexist, and the role of diet is vital. Eating a nutritionally rich diet with adequate calories and protein and a full range of vitamins and minerals – especially vitamin C and zinc – has been shown to improve wound healing. Being well nourished also protects the integrity of your skin and guards against breakdown. If you're at risk of or recovering from a pressure sore, your doctor may prescribe vitamin C and zinc supplements, which you can find at health food stores and most pharmacies. Patients with pressure ulcers may require higher protein diets and more energy than other bedridden patients do. Zinc supplementation is often promoted as aiding in wound healing, yet evidence for its efficacy is far from conclusive.

What are the main infectious and non-infectious causes of systemic inflammatory response syndrome?

Systemic inflammatory response syndrome (SIRS) is an inflammatory state of the body, without a proven source of infection, which occurs when inflammatory mediators are released into the systemic circulation. Sepsis, SIRS and multiple organ dysfunction syndrome (MODS) represent the progressive stages of the same illnesses. The causes of SIRS are categorised as being either infectious or non-infectious. Although infection can be a common cause of SIRS, it is not the only one. There are also different non-infectious causes, such as severe trauma and complications of surgery, acute pancreatitis, burns, haematoma and venous thrombosis, pulmonary and myocardial infarction, acute adrenal insufficiency, increased cytokine release, neuroleptic malignant syndrome, lymphoma, hypernephroma, tumour lysis syndrome, drug overdose and immunodeficiency (e.g. AIDS).

What is the most appropriate diet for systemic inflammatory response syndrome?

The role of diet and especially of immunonutrition in critically ill patients is vital, though still controversial. Enteral feedings with arginine, glutamine and omega-3 fatty acids and supplementation with nucleotides have been shown to be beneficial for these patients. Thus, a diet enriched with eicosapentaenoic acid (EPA), gamma-linolenic acid (GLA) and elevated antioxidants may contribute to better hospital outcomes and is associated with lower mortality rates. The appropriate provision of these nutrients has been shown to decrease infectious complications, the duration of hospitalisation and of mechanical ventilation. The type of feeding formula and the route of nutrition vary, according mainly to the aetiology of SIRS.

What is the role of nutritional support in the treatment of multiple organ dysfunction syndrome?

MODS, also known as multiple organ failure (MOF), is a condition characterised by severe systemic inflammation and caused by altered organ function in acutely ill patients. The major causes of MODS are trauma, burns, haemorrhage, autoimmune disease and over-dosage of drugs and toxic chemicals. Nosocomial infections – related to decreased immune function and gut-barrier malfunction, increased catabolism, morbidity and high rates of mortality – are the most common problems in critically ill patients with MODS. MOF is the leading cause of mortality (50–80% of all deaths) in surgical ICUs. Enteral feeding in MODS patients is the preferred route of nutrition, while the addition of nutritional substrates, such as glutamine, seems to preserve intestinal mucosal integrity and lymphoid tissue in the gastrointestinal tract, decreasing intestinal permeability and bacterial translocation.

Further reading

Berger MM (2006) Antioxidant micronutrients in major trauma and burns: Evidence and practice. *Nutrition in Clinical Practice* **21**(5): 438–49.

Collis N, Smith G, Fenton OM (1999) Accuracy of burn size estimation and subsequent fluid resuscitation prior to arrival at the Yorkshire Regional Burns Unit: A three year retrospective study. *Burns* **25**(4): 345–51.

Darbar A (2001) Nutritional requirements in severe head injury. *Nutrition* **17**(1): 71–2.

Dickerson R (2002) Estimating energy and protein requirements of thermally injured patients: Art or science? *Nutrition* **18**(5): 439–42.

Fodor L, Fodor A, Ramon Y *et al.* (2005) Controversies in fluid resuscitation for burn management: Literature review and our experience. *Injury* **37**(5): 374–9.

Katherine J, Desneves BE, Todorovic AC, Crowe TC (2005) Treatment with supplementary arginine, vitamin C and zinc in patients with pressure ulcers: A randomised controlled trial. *Clinical Nutrition* **24**(6): 979–87.

Lee SK, Posthauer ME, Dorner B *et al.* (2006) Pressure ulcer healing with a concentrated, fortified, collagen protein hydrolysate supplement: A randomized controlled trial. *Advances in Skin & Wound Care* **19**(2): 92–6.

Marik PE, Zaloga GP (2008) Immunonutrition in critically ill patients: A systematic review and analysis of the literature. *Intensive Care Medicine* **34**(11): 1980–90.

Masters B, Wood F (2008) Nutrition support in burns: Is there consistency in practice? *Journal of Burn Care & Research* **29**(4): 561–71.

Megan Boitano (2006) Hypocaloric feeding of the critically ill. *Nutrition in Clinical Practice* **21**(6): 617–22.

Milner S, Mottar R, Smith Ch (2001) The burn wheel: An innovative method for calculating the need for fluid resuscitation in burned patients. *American Journal of Nursing* **101**(11): 35–7.

Parke AL, Liu PT, Parke DV (2003) Multiple organ dysfunction syndrome. *Inflammopharmacology* **11**(1): 87–95.

Perel P, Edwards P, Wentz R, Roberts I (2006) Systematic review of prognostic models in traumatic brain injury. *BMC: Medical Informatics and Decision Making* **14**(6): 38.

Spindler-Vesel A, Bengmark S *et al.* (2007) Synbiotics, prebiotics, glutamine, or peptide in early enteral nutrition: A randomized study in trauma patients. *Journal of Parenteral and Enteral Nutrition* **31**(2): 119–26.

Wasiak J, Cleland H, Jeffery R (2007) Early versus late enteral nutritional support in adults with burn injury: A systematic review. *Journal of Human Nutrition and Dietetics* **20**(2): 75–83.

Waxman K, Rebello T, Pinderski L *et al.* (1987) Protein loss across burn wounds. *Journal of Trauma* **27**(2): 136.

Winkler MF, Ainsley MM (2004) Medical nutrition therapy for metabolic stress: Sepsis, trauma, burns, and surgery. In: Mahan LK, Escott-Stump S (eds), *Krause's Food, Nutrition, and Diet Therapy*, (11th edn), WB Saunders, Philadelphia, pp. 1059–76.

Wischmeyer PE (2008) Glutamine: Role in critical illness and ongoing clinical trials. *Current Opinion in Gastroenterology* **24**(2): 190–7.

Chapter 13

Neoplastic Diseases

Meropi Kontogianni

What lifestyle recommendations are important for cancer prevention?

In 2007, the World Cancer Research Fund and the American Institute of Cancer Research published a global perspective on food, nutrition, physical activity and the prevention of cancer. Table 13.1 describes the main recommendations of this report.

In what ways can cancer affect nutritional status?

Cancer has a profound impact on patients' physical functions, psychological well-being and social life. Depending upon the site of the cancer, digestion and absorption of nutrients may be disturbed (e.g. owing to diarrhoea, malabsorption). Additionally, their metabolism may be altered. Proteolysis and lipolysis are accelerated, while muscle protein synthesis is depressed, resulting in a loss of lean body mass and fat tissue. Additionally, carbohydrate metabolism is modified by tumour growth (e.g. the hepatic glucose production and Cori cycle activity are increased while the insulin sensitivity of peripheral tissues is reduced). These alterations contribute to an increase in energy expenditure and may result in progressive wasting.

However, in spite of hypermetabolism and weight loss (exacerbated by stress, pain, infection, surgical procedures), patients' food intake is usually not increased, thus further promoting wasting. Furthermore, cancer cachexia – characterised by weight loss, reduction of fat and lean body masses, anorexia with reduced food intake, early satiety, dysgeusia, dysphagia, fatigue, anaemia, hypoalbuminaemia, progressive debilitation – also deteriorates nutritional status. Nonetheless, besides the physical effects of cancer, patients are often suffering from psychological disturbances as well, and

Table 13.1 World Cancer Research Fund/American Institute of Cancer Research recommendations on cancer prevention.

Recommendation 1: **Body Fatness**
Be as lean as possible within the normal range (according to WHO or national governments) of body weight.
● Avoid weight gain and increases in waist circumference throughout adulthood

Recommendation 2: **Physical Activity**
Be physically active as part of everyday life (brisk walking for at least 30 minutes/day.
● As fitness improves, increase to 60 minutes or more of moderate or to 30 minutes or more of vigorous physical activity/day.

Recommendation 3: **Foods and drinks that promote weight gain**
Limit consumption of energy-dense foods (energy content >225-275 kcal/100 g).
● Average energy density of diets should be lowered towards 125 kcal/100 g.
● Avoid sugary drinks (mostly those with added sugars; however, fruit juices should be also limited).

Recommendation 4: **Plant foods**
Eat mostly foods of plant origin.
● Population average consumption of non-starchy vegetables and fruits should be at least 600 g (21 oz) daily. Individuals should consume at least five portions/servings (i.e. 400 g or 14 oz) of a variety of non-starchy vegetables and fruits per day.
● Eat relatively unprocessed cereals (grains) and/or pulses (legumes) with every meal. Limit refined cereals.

Recommendation 5: **Animal foods**
Limit intake of red meat (beef, pork, lamb and goat) and avoid processed meat (meat preserved by smoking, curing or salting or addition of chemical preservatives).
● Population average consumption of red meat should be no more than 300 g (11 oz) per week.
● Goal for the individual is consumption of less than 500 g (18 oz) per week of red meat and very little if any to be processed.

Recommendation 6: **Alcoholic drinks**
Limit alcoholic drinks.
● If alcoholic drinks are consumed, limit consumption to no more than two drinks/day for men and one drink a day for women (one drink = 10–15 g of ethanol).
● Children and pregnant women should not consume alcoholic drinks.

Recommendation 7: **Preservation, processing, preparation**
Limit consumption of salt. Avoid mouldy cereals or pulses (aflatoxin contamination risk).
● Population average consumption of salt from all sources should be less than 5 g (2 g of sodium) per day.
● On an individual basis salt consumption should be limited to less than 6 g (2.4 g of sodium) per day.
● Methods of preservation that do not or need not use salt include refrigeration, freezing, drying, bottling, canning and fermentation.

Recommendation 8: **Dietary supplements**
Aim to meet nutritional needs through diet alone. In some cases of illness or dietary inadequacy, supplements may be valuable. Dietary supplements are not recommended for cancer prevention.

Special recommendation 1: **Breastfeeding**
Mothers to breastfeed; children to be breastfed.
● Aim to breastfeed infants exclusively up to six months and continue with complementary feeding thereafter.

Special recommendation 2: **Cancer survivors**
Follow the recommendations for cancer prevention.

---

particularly depression, whereas oncology treatment such as surgery, chemotherapy and radiotherapy produce additional acute and chronic symptoms which increase energy expenditure and jeopardise food intake (e.g. by changes in taste, dry mouth, nausea, vomiting) and nutritional status.

What are the main characteristics of cancer cachexia? How does it affect the patient's prognosis?

The cancer cachexia syndrome, characterised by marked weight loss, anorexia, asthenia and anaemia, is invariably associated with the presence and growth of the tumour and leads to a malnutrition status owing to the induction of anorexia or decreased food intake. In addition, the competition for nutrients between the tumour and the host leads to an accelerated starvation state that promotes severe metabolic disturbances in the host, including hypermetabolism, which leads to decreased energetic efficiency. The predominant manifestation of cancer cachexia is the steadily progressive depletion of muscle mass, which is not substantially reversible with any of the currently available nutritional, metabolic or pharmacological approaches. Cancer cachexia mainly results from circulating factors produced by the tumour or by the host's immune system in response to the tumour, such as cytokines released by lymphocytes and/or monocytes/macrophages. A number of pro-inflammatory cytokines, including interleukin (IL)-1, IL-6, tumour necrosis factor (TNF)-α, interferon (IFN)-α and IFN-γ, have been implicated in the pathogenesis of cachexia associated with human cancer.

The complications associated with the appearance of the cachexia syndrome affect both the physiological and biochemical balance of the patient and influence the efficiency of anticancer treatment, resulting in a considerably decreased survival time. At the metabolic level, cachexia is associated with the loss of body lipid stores. Alterations in lipid metabolism are partially mediated by changes in circulating hormone concentrations (insulin, glucagon and glucocorticoids, in particular) or in their effectiveness. However, a large number of observations point towards cytokines, polypeptides released mainly by immune cells, as the molecules responsible for the above-mentioned metabolic derangements. The most important carbohydrate abnormalities are insulin resistance, increased glucose synthesis, gluconeogenesis and Cori cycle activity, and decreased glucose tolerance and turnover. The main pathological changes of protein metabolism include increased protein turnover, muscle catabolism, and liver and tumour protein synthesis, while muscle protein synthesis is decreased. The main abnormalities found in lipid metabolism are enhanced lipid mobilisation, decreased lipogenesis, decreased lipoprotein lipase activity, elevated triglycerides and decreased high-density lipoproteins, increased venous glycerol and decreased glycerol clearance from the plasma. Box 13.1 describes the main consequences of cancer cachexia.

Chapter 13

> **Box 13.1** Main consequences of cancer cachexia syndrome.
>
> - Impaired quality of life.
> - Reduced response to chemotherapy.
> - Increased risk of chemotherapy-induced toxicity.
> - Impaired immune competence.
> - Reduced performance status and muscle function.
> - Increased risk of postoperative complications.
> - Longer hospital stay.
> - Higher prescription and consultation rates.
> - Shorter survival time.

What are the energy and protein requirements of cancer patients?

Cancer itself does not have a consistent effect on resting energy expenditure (REE). Oncological treatment, however, may modulate energy expenditure. REE can be unchanged, increased or decreased in relation to the predicted energy expenditure. The energy requirements of cancer patients should therefore be assumed to be normal unless there are specific data showing otherwise. If REE cannot be measured in individual cases then assumption of total energy expenditure (TEE) calculated from equations is acceptable. As a rule of thumb, the following assumptions for TEE can be made for non-obese patients using the actual body weight:

- ambulant patients: 30–35 kcal/kg body weight/day
- bedridden patients: 20–25 kcal/kg body weight/day

These assumptions are less accurate for severely underweight (actual TEE per kg is higher in this group) and for severely overweight subjects (actual TEE per kg is lower). With regard to protein needs, the optimal nitrogen supply for cancer patients cannot be easily determined. Recommendations range from a minimum protein supply of 1 g/kg body weight/day to a target supply of 1.2–2 g/kg body weight/day.

How can radiotherapy affect dietary intake?

The effect of radiotherapy on a patient's nutritional status depends on the extent of body area irradiated, as well as the type, quantity and duration of radiotherapy and the individual's response. Gastrointestinal mucosa is highly vulnerable to radiation therapy, with the common emetic adverse effects having an obvious impact on food intake. Radiation therapy also has a direct toxic effect on the taste buds of the tongue and their innervating nerve fibres, as well as on the microvilli of the gastrointestinal mucosa; it can impair secretory cell functions, resulting in a reduction of output and an alteration in the viscosity of saliva. Radiation therapy to the head and neck region, including cancer of the mouth, tongue, salivary glands, throat and face, has been associated with anorexia, oesophagitis, xerostomia, nausea, vomiting, dysphagia, odynophagia, sore throat, alterations in taste and smell and trismus, all of which can significantly reduce food intake and negatively affect a patient's nutritional status. Therefore, in these cases regular nutritional assessment is very important.

Moreover, radiation to the abdomen or pelvic area, including cancer of the cervix, colon, rectum, pancreas and prostate, may cause acute diarrhoea, anorexia, nausea, vomiting, abdominal pain, enteritis and colitis, and in severe cases ulceration and perforation, owing to irradiation damage of the gastrointestinal mucosa. Another complication of radiation therapy, which can have a profound long-term effect on nutritional status, is chronic radiation enteropathy. This can cause severe, multiple gastrointestinal strictures and fistulas, leading to significant nutritional deficiencies and malnutrition. Nutritional assessment and advice from an experienced dietitian may alleviate symptoms and cover patients' nutritional needs. Radiation-induced diarrhoea may require some changes in the patient's diet, the most common of which are reduction in fibre, fat or lactose.

What are the main nutrition-related side effects of chemotherapy?

The nutrition-related side effects associated with chemotherapy depend on the regime and dose prescribed. Each drug has different side effects, most of which may affect appetite and food intake, including nausea and vomiting, taste changes, stomatitis, mucositis with consequent sore or painful mouth, oesophagitis, diarrhoea and constipation. Table 13.2 refers to common dietetic advice for the treatment of the above-mentioned problems that affect food intake.

How can bacterial contamination in food be minimised for immunosuppressed patients?

Treatment of leukaemia and other haematological malignancies often involves bone marrow or peripheral blood cell transplantation and requires patient immunosuppression. During immunosuppression, foods that are generally contraindicated are those which are uncooked or have been exposed to air and hence likely to be contaminated with bacteria or fungi. Immunosuppressed patients should therefore avoid:

- raw or undercooked meat, fish, shellfish, eggs or unpasteurised milk, processed meats like salami and paté, sushi, 'live' or 'bio' yoghurt, soft cheeses (e.g. Brie, Camembert, cottage cheese, Roquefort), mayonnaise.
- raw vegetables and fruits with skins or which are partially damaged.

Chapter 13

Table 13.2 Basic dietary advice for chemotherapy side effects[a].

Side effect	Dietary manipulation
Loss of appetite	• Consume small and frequent meals, when appetite is best. • Serve food in manageable portions. The sight of large portions is off-putting. • Eat slowly, chew well and relax between courses and after a meal. • Eat anything that is particularly fancied. • Do not consume large quantities of liquids before or during meals. • A short walk before a meal may help appetite. • If alcohol is allowed small quantities before or during a meal can stimulate appetite. • Avoid exposure to cooking smells during food preparation.
Loss of taste	• Choose foods full of flavour and aroma. • Use seasonings (e.g. vinaigrette), herbs (e.g. basil, oregano, garlic), spices (e.g. curry, pepper, sweet paprika), lemon juice to enhance flavour. • Lemon juice in water before food may be helpful. • Marinating food in wine, beer, cider or fruit juice may also enhance flavour.
Changes in taste	• Avoid any food with an unpleasant taste. • Allow hot food to cool before eating since high temperature enhances unpleasant taste. • If meat tastes unpleasant, consume other sources of high biological value proteins. Try to marinate meat or consume cold. • If you experience a metallic taste, a small portion of lemon juice in water before eating may help.
Xerostomia (dry mouth)	• Moisten meals by adding sauces, seasonings, gravy, cream or evaporated milk. • Avoid grilling or frying as cooking methods and prefer others that maintain moisture (e.g. pressure cooking, steaming, boiling). • Avoid dry/rough foods (e.g. toasts, biscuits, crackers, cereal bars, crisps). • Sip liquids during meals. • Prefer sharp-tasting foods (e.g. those flavoured with lemon, grapefruit and rhubarb).
Sore or painful mouth	• Eat soft, moist foods. • Avoid very dry or rough-textured foods (see above). • Avoid salty or spicy foods. • Avoid orange, grapefruit and lemon juice, as well as vinegar.

[a] For management of nausea, vomiting, constipation and diarrhoea, see Chapter 7.

- foods in opened containers or shared by others (e.g. large cartons of ice cream, jars of jam, bottled sauces).
- foods that are approaching their 'use by' date.
- cooking methods such as microwave or cook-chill systems and barbecued food.
- reheating already heated food and refreezing thawed frozen foods.
- storing raw and cooked food together.
- eating and drinking away from home.

Is enteral nutrition indicated for cancer patients?

The aetiology of malnutrition in patients with cancer is multifactorial. Impaired caloric intake, altered metabolism and an increased inflammatory response all contribute. However, impaired caloric intake due to gastrointestinal failure is the most important factor. Enteral nutrition is a critical therapy for treating malnutrition associated with cancer and is indicated in any malnourished patient with a functional gastrointestinal tract who is unable to ingest sufficient nutrients orally, as long as enteral access can safely be achieved. Enteral nutrition is preferred over parenteral nutrition because it is more physiological, simpler, safer and less costly. Common indications include dysphagia due to head and neck cancer, oesophageal obstruction, gastric outlet obstruction or critical illness requiring prolonged mechanical ventilation. Moreover, in patients experiencing anorexia or aversion to certain food groups (e.g. meat), oral nutritional supplements may help achieve required energy and protein intakes.

With regard to type of enteral formula, over the past several years, formulas designed to modulate the immune response have been developed and have been suggested for use in the patient with cancer. Various nutrients, including arginine, glutamine, omega-3 fatty acids and polyribonucleotide (RNA), have been shown to alter the immune response. To date, several prospective, randomised studies evaluating the effect of these formulas on patients with cancer have been performed. Although some studies have shown a decrease in infectious complications, none has shown a statistically significant survival benefit.

According to the European Society of Clinical Nutrition and Metabolism (ESPEN), randomised, clinical trial evidence concerning the use of formulas rich in omega-3 in cancer patients is contradictory/controversial, and at present it is not possible to reach any firm conclusion with regard to any improvement in nutritional status/physical function. In addition, it is unlikely that omega-3 fatty acids prolong survival in advanced cancer. However, in all cancer patients undergoing major abdominal surgery, ESPEN recommends preoperative enteral nutrition, preferably with immune modulating substrates for 5–7 days independent of a patient's nutritional status. For other cancer patients who may need enteral nutrition administration either in the form of oral supplements or via tube feeding, a standard polymeric formula covers their nutritional needs.

Chapter 13

Further reading

Arends J, Bodoky G, Bozzetti F *et al.* (2006) ESPEN guidelines on enteral nutrition: Non-surgical oncology. *Clinical Nutrition* **25**(2): 245–59.

Marín Caro MM, Laviano A, Pichard C (2007) Nutritional intervention and quality of life in adult oncology patients. *Clinical Nutrition* **26**(3): 289–301.

Pattison AJ (1993) Review of current practice in 'clean' diets in the UK. *Journal of Human Nutrition and Dietetics* **6**(1): 3–11.

Schattner M (2003) Enteral nutritional support of the patient with cancer: Route and role. *Journal of Clinical Gastroenterology* **36**(4): 297–302.

Thomas B (2007) *Manual of Dietetic Practice*, (3rd edn). Blackwell Science Ltd, Oxford.

Van Cutsem E, Arends J (2005) The causes and consequences of cancer-associated malnutrition. *European Journal of Oncology Nursing* **9**(suppl. 2): S51–63.

World Cancer Research Fund, American Institute of Cancer Research (2007) *Food, Nutrition, Physical Activity, and the Prevention of Cancer: A global perspective.* AICR, Washington.

Chapter 14

Rheumatic Diseases

Meropi Kontogianni

Osteoporosis

What are the main nutritional goals for the prevention and treatment of osteoporosis?

The main nutritional goals for the prevention and treatment of osteoporosis are:

- adequate intake of calcium and vitamin D throughout life stages
- adequate intake of protein according to dietary reference intake
- avoidance of excessive phosphorous ingestion (calcium/phosphorus ratio = 1:1 ideally)
- diet rich in fruits and vegetables
- avoidance of excessive sodium intake; an intake of about 2400 mg per day is not detrimental
- caffeine intake should be limited in individuals who do not reach recommended calcium intake; otherwise, an intake of three cups of coffee per day does not impose a negative effect on bone metabolism
- limit alcohol intake to 8–30 ml (0.28–1.055 fl oz) per day; during childhood and adolescence, alcohol should be completely avoided, because it affects peak bone mass in a negative way.

What dietary factors decrease calcium bioavailability?

The excessive daily intake of phosphorus, sodium, caffeine or alcohol increases mainly calcium excretion and therefore reduces its availability in the body. Moreover, phytates (e.g. in wholegrain and pulses) and oxalates (e.g. in spinach and rhubarb) in foods bind calcium in the food per se and reduce its absorption significantly. Finally, excessive fibre intake (40–50 g/day) reduces calcium enteral absorption.

Are dairy products the major source of calcium in the diet?

Calcium is present in a wide range of foods, but not all of these are good sources of calcium, since the calcium that they contain may not be well absorbed, as described in the previous paragraph. Dairy products, such as milk, yoghurt and cheese, are all plentiful sources of well-absorbed calcium and, in Western countries, dairy products supply up to two-thirds of total calcium intake. Fish which is consumed with the soft edible bones (such as whitebait, canned sardines or canned salmon) is also a good source of calcium, and in some countries several foods are fortified with calcium (e.g. in the UK, there is a statutory requirement that flour is fortified with calcium). Alternative sources of calcium, such as cruciferous vegetables (e.g. cauliflower, cabbage, Brussels sprouts), fortified industry products or calcium supplements become very important in the case of people having problems with the ingestion of dairy products (e.g. lactose intolerance, milk allergy or for vegans). In addition, recent studies on calcium absorption from mineral waters showed an absorption rate similar to that of milk (~30%) and a careful choice of a mineral water rich in calcium can contribute significantly to one's daily calcium intake. Table 14.1 presents common food sources of calcium and its fractional absorption.

Table 14.1 Common food sources of calcium and its fractional absorption.

Food[a]	Serving size (g)	Calcium content (mg)	Fractional absorption (%)	Servings needed to equal 240 ml milk
Milk	240	300	32.1	1.0
Dry-roasted almonds	28	80	21.2	5.7
Beans, red	172	40.5	17.0	14.0
Beans, white	110	113	17.0	5.0
Broccoli	71	35	52.6	5.2
Brussels sprouts	78	19	63.8	8.0
Cabbage green	75	25	64.9	5.9
Cauliflower	62	17	68.6	8.2
Kale	65	47	58.8	3.5
Radish	50	14	74.4	9.2
Sesame seeds, no hulls	28	37	20.8	12.2
Soya milk	120	5	31.0	60.4
Spinach	90	122	5.1	15.5
Tofu, calcium set	126	258	31.0	1.2
Turnip greens	72	99	51.6	1.9
Watercress	17	20	67.0	7.2

[a]Based on $1/2$ cup serving size except for milk and sesame/almonds seeds (1 oz.).
Data adapted from Weaver CM, Plawecki KL (1994) Dietary calcium: Adequacy of a vegetarian diet. *American Journal of Clinical Nutrition* **59**(suppl. 5): S1238–41.

How important is the dietary intake of vitamin D?

Diet is considered a secondary source of vitamin D, since only a few foods contain appreciable amounts. The vitamin D requirement for most human beings (90–100%) can come from exposure to sunlight. However, the latitude, season, way of living (mainly staying or working indoors) and the widespread use of sunscreen creams significantly affect the exposure to ultraviolet B (UVB) radiation, which is necessary for conversion of the vitamin D precursor in the skin to active vitamin D. Today, Vitamin D deficiency is an epidemic in many populations, not only in older people but also commonly in prepubescent children, adolescents and young and middle-aged adults and has insidious consequences for the skeleton. Given the fact that Vitamin D deficiency is very common, food sources become more important.

The richest dietary sources of vitamin D are oily fish, such as herring, mackerel and sardines, eggs, meat, meat products and offal. Fortification of popular drinks like milk and orange juice, as well as of margarines and spreads, breakfast cereals and milk powder seems to be imperative, even in sunny countries.

Does vegetarianism affect bone health?

The bone health of vegetarians has been a topic of interest for many years, but few data are available. Calcium intake in lacto-vegetarians is similar to that in non-vegetarians, whereas vegans usually have a substantially lower calcium intake unless they consume a lot of calcium-rich plant foods, such as cruciferous vegetables. Both high-protein consumption (particularly without supporting calcium/alkali intakes) and low-protein intakes (particularly in vegan diets) have been shown to be detrimental to the skeleton. It has been suggested that the absence of meat may be beneficial for bone health because of a reduced 'acid load', but whether this factor is important remains to be seen. Moreover, there is growing support from a combination of clinical, observational and intervention studies for the beneficial effect of fruit and vegetable intake on bone health. The mechanisms behind this 'fruit and veg' link remain to be fully determined: these foods provide not only a source of dietary alkali (for which there is more and more data to suggest a critical role for the skeleton in acid-base homeostasis) but also a wide variety of micronutrients, many of which may have an effect on bone.

Overall, it is not clear whether the bone health of vegetarians is better or worse than that of comparable non-vegetarians. Early results from the EPIC-Oxford study show no difference in fracture rates between vegetarians and non-vegetarians, but do show the importance of adequate calcium intake in reducing fracture risk.

What is the impact of weight and weight loss on bone mass?

A low body weight is associated with low bone mass and an increased risk of fractures, whereas obesity is associated with increased bone mass and

Chapter 14

reduced bone turnover and loss. Although the additional bone mass in obese compared with lean subjects contributes only to ~0.5 kg (1.1 lb) of total body weight, it contributes to ~20% of total bone mineral content, thus making a substantial contribution to the higher risk of osteoporosis in lean compared with obese subjects.

Some studies show that a 10% weight loss results in ~1–2% bone loss at various bone sites. In addition, other studies have shown that there is greater bone loss (>1%) with weight loss in normal weight [less than ~60 kg (132 lb)] compared to overweight or obese individuals (<1% bone loss). Importantly, weight loss and weight-cycling throughout adulthood and older age were shown to increase hip fracture risk. Losing as little as 5% of body weight increases the fracture risk in postmenopausal women, especially in those who are relatively thin in middle age, as well as in older men. Groups vulnerable to bone loss due to weight reduction will likely benefit from a higher calcium intake and/or possibly higher levels of vitamin D intake or other nutrients. An individualised diet programme to minimise bone changes is suggested for all persons, but especially for those ≥50 years old in combination with mild resistance exercise sessions under medical supervision. Unnecessary weight loss efforts throughout life, especially in adolescents and in women generally, should be discouraged since they impose a detrimental effect on bone mass.

In what ways do fractures affect a patient's nutritional needs?

Patients with a fracture, especially in the hip region, are commonly malnourished, which significantly affects their outcome and recovery. A fracture is a trauma that increases patients' basic metabolic rate; however, patients do not need large amounts of energy, since their physical activity is limited during the recovery phase. In general, an energy intake of 30 kcal/kg body weight (276.3 kJ/lb body weight) covers the needs of most patients. Additionally, protein needs are increased, as in all traumas. Patients with fracture risks need at least 1.2 g/kg (0.55 g/lb) body weight of protein, unless there is another health problem that does not allow high protein intakes. Studies of the effect of routine nutritional supplementation in fracture patients suggest that the strongest evidence exists for oral protein and energy feeds, but the evidence is still very weak and needs further investigation. Patients with fractures also need a supplemented dose of calcium (1000–1200 mg/day) and vitamin D (800 IU/day) to help recovery and prevent another fracture.

Commonly, patients with fractures are at high risk of developing pressure ulcers; if this happens, nutritional needs are modulated as follows:

- Try to correct the underfed state by arranging a well-balanced daily diet by the sufficient provision of calories [30–35 kcal/kg (57–66.6 kJ/lb)] and protein [1.0–1.5 g/kg (0.45–0.68 g/lb)].
- Sufficient fluid intake [1 ml/kcal (0.14 fl oz/kJ) or 30 ml/kg (0.48 fl oz/lb)] in order to prevent dehydration.
- Nutritional supplements containing arginine, vitamins C, A, E, thiamine and zinc may help in healing the pressure ulcer.

Gout

What dietary factors affect uric acid levels and/or worsen the symptoms of gout?

Various purine-rich foods and a high-protein intake have been traditionally considered risk factors for gout, but the associations had not been prospectively confirmed. According to recent large prospective cohorts, higher levels of meat and seafood consumption are associated with an increased risk of gout, whereas a higher level of consumption of dairy products is associated with a decreased risk. Moderate intake of purine-rich vegetables (e.g. tomatoes, mushrooms, spinach, asparagus, cauliflower) or protein of phytic origin (e.g. from beans, peas) is not associated with an increased risk of gout. Ethanol intake has been shown to increase serum uric acid level via both decreased urate excretion and increased production. Beer and liquor have been found to raise serum uric acid, whereas results from epidemiological studies suggest that moderate consumption of wine may not increase serum uric acid levels, as do other alcoholic beverages.

The general dietary advice for people at risk of hyperuricaemia or gout is the restriction of organ meats (liver, kidneys, sweetbreads), meat extracts, consommé, gravies, as well as anchovies, sardines in oil, fish roes, herring. In addition a protein intake close to the recommended, moderation in the consumption of not only beer but also other forms of alcohol and consumption of 8 to 16 cups of fluid/day, at least half as water, are essential. In the obese, controlled weight management has the potential to lower serum urate in a quantitatively similar way to relatively unpalatable 'low purine' diets.

Autoimmune rheumatoid diseases

Is nutrition a predisposing factor for autoimmune rheumatoid diseases?

Many researchers subscribe to the theory that the long-term consumption of foods with pro-inflammatory properties, such as meat and the abstention from foods with anti-inflammatory properties, such as fish, fruits and vegetables, may promote the development of autoimmune diseases. However, scientific data have, so far, not managed to reveal such a relationship and attribute the predisposition to autoimmune diseases to other factors, namely genetic, hormonal, environmental or psychological.

How does rheumatoid arthritis affect body composition?

Rheumatoid cachexia was first described over a century ago. However, this 'bad condition' has been recognised as a common problem among patients with rheumatoid arthritis (RA) relatively recently. While cachexia generally connotes a state of advanced malnutrition and wasting, we now know that this term refers, more specifically, to a loss of body cell mass (BCM).

Chapter 14

TNF-alpha and IL-1-beta, which play the most important role in the patho-genesis of RA, affect total body protein significantly, by promoting protein breakdown and loss. Loss of BCM greater than 40% of baseline is associ-ated with death. However, even with as little as 5% loss of BCM, there are demonstrable changes in morbidity, including loss of muscle strength, altered energy metabolism and increased susceptibility to infections.

Rheumatoid cachexia should be viewed as an important contributor to in-creased morbidity and premature mortality in RA and in two-thirds of patients is combined with obesity, and the state has been described as 'rheumatoid cachectic obesity'. Patients with RA usually present with increased fat depo-sition throughout the body, apart from in the legs; therefore, fat distribution becomes more central, and this is more prominent in patients receiving cor-ticosteroids for long periods. In addition, low habitual physical activity has consistently been observed in RA and is an important consequence of, and contributor to, muscle wasting. Moreover, low physical activity predisposes to fat gain and is believed to precipitate a negative reinforcing cycle of muscle loss, reduced physical function and fat gain in RA, which leads to 'cachectic obesity'.

Bone mineral density in several sites is also reduced in patients with RA, compared to healthy controls. This finding has been attributed to several factors, namely long-term corticosteroid use, low physical activity level, in-creased secretion of TNF-alpha and IL-1-beta which promote osteoclast differentiation and, additionally, the low intake of calcium and vitamin D. Therefore, any nutritional assessment of patients with RA should always focus on the dietary intake of these nutrients.

What are the aims of nutritional treatment in patients with rheumatoid arthritis?

The main dietary goals for patients with RA are:

- muscle mass preservation, through appropriate diet, especially in terms of protein intake, and exercise counselling
- prevention of fat mass increase, especially at central body parts
- emphasis on all the nutrients that optimise bone health (calcium, vitamin D, protein) and restriction of those with a detrimental effect (salt, alcohol, vitamin A)
- diet adaptation according to medication (especially during corticosteroid use)
- modification of diet texture according to chewing, swallowing and self-feeding ability.

Do elimination diets have a role in the treatment of rheumatoid arthritis?

Patients with RA often claim that their symptoms are alleviated by special di-ets or by simply eliminating certain foods, and it has been proposed that food-related antigens, predominantly from protein sources, may provoke hypersensitivity responses, which may increase symptoms of RA. Controlled studies, involving the exclusion of foods such as red meat, dairy products, cereals and wheat gluten foods, have reported inconsistent results, with either improvements or no change in subjective and objective measures of symptoms. Furthermore, evidence exists that RA is a Th1-dominated autoimmune disease, while allergic reactions are mediated by Th2 cells and their related cytokines (i.e. IL-4, IL-10), and it is estimated that probably less than 5% of RA patients do have an actual immune sensitivity to specific foods, which is similar to the level found in the general population. These facts and recently published papers dealing with the question of food intolerance in RA contradicted a significant role of allergic reactions in the pathophysiology of the majority of RA patients.

Elimination diets are usually preceded by a period of fasting, which may confound the reported improvement in symptoms. Fasting is known to suppress inflammation. The mechanism by which this operates is not completely understood, but may involve a reduction in the release of pro-inflammatory cytokines, reduced leukotriene formation and altered intestinal permeability, which may decrease the penetration of immunostimulants from the intestines. Short-term fasting with or without a prolonged vegetarian diet may represent another interesting dietary approach in RA. The clinical effectiveness of this dietary approach, however, remains unknown, and possible anti-inflammatory mechanisms are far from understood. Fasting, elimination and elemental diets cannot be regarded as having an established place in treatment but may help individual patients. Their use needs to be assessed by sequential withdrawal and rechallenged, with formal documentation of subjective and objective parameters. Patients with RA should be discouraged from undertaking self-imposed elimination diets, which may compromise their nutritional status and should be advised to eat a well-balanced diet, according to their anthropometric and clinical characteristics and the medication they receive.

What should a dietitian bear in mind about the nutrition of a patient with systemic erythematosus lupus?

Patients with systemic erythematosus lupus (SEL) may present several and various symptoms, according to the affected organ or systems of the body. The most common nutrition-related complications of SEL are lupus nephritis, which is accompanied with urinary protein loss and electrolyte disturbances, hypertension and atherosclerosis. Therefore, each patient, according to their symptoms and problems, may follow a different diet. The dietitian should monitor patients' biochemical indices and symptoms and change the diet accordingly. Moreover, a patient's medication should be carefully monitored since it may influence the diet regime.

What dietary modifications are necessary for the management of xerostomia in patients with Sjögren syndrome?

Restriction of carbohydrates, especially of the simple ones like sugar and honey, as well as of the food and commercially available products that contain them, can help patients with xerostomia. Moreover, hard and dehydrated food (e.g. rusks, Melba toast, crackers) or food at extreme temperatures should be avoided. Conversely, frequent cleaning of the teeth and the use of mouthwash are common practices that the patient could find helpful and should always bear in mind.

Which of the drugs used for the treatment of rheumatic diseases can cause drug–nutrient interactions or impose certain dietary modifications?

Corticosteroids are the cornerstone of treatment for several rheumatic diseases; however, their long-term use may generate several adverse effects, some of which will affect the patient's diet. In order to avoid severe fluid retention when using corticosteroids, patients should follow a low-sodium diet. Moreover, corticosteroids may raise blood sugar or even cholesterol levels, and therefore patients should be advised to restrict the consumption of simple sugars or saturated fat, respectively. If a patient's blood glucose level rises significantly, they should restrict themselves to a diabetic diet while they are taking corticosteroids. In addition, since corticosteroids induce protein catabolism, patients should consume the necessary daily protein amount and should achieve an optimum dietary intake in terms of bone health, since long-term corticosteroid use comprises an important risk factor for osteoporosis. Therefore, during corticosteroid treatment, it is vital to ensure the recommended calcium and vitamin D intake, either from foods or from supplements. Patients receiving large doses of corticosteroids usually report a weight gain, and this can be attributed entirely to the increase in appetite that the drug causes. Dietitians should inform their patients of this side effect and encourage them to follow a certain diet according to their energy needs and consumption and not according to their appetite.

Methotrexate is a known antagonist of folic acid, and folic acid levels may be reduced in patients receiving this drug. The careful monitoring of folic acid levels is required, whereas a low weekly supplementation dose of folic acid (<5 mg) can prevent deficiency of this nutrient. Dietitians should bear in mind that patients receiving cyclosporin should completely avoid the consumption of grapefruit and its juice, since this fruit contains a factor that increases the drug's toxicity.

Can patients with rheumatic diseases benefit from alternative medicine supplements?

There are several over-the-counter dietary supplements, herbs or combinations of nutrients and herbs either from large reliable industries or from other, less safe, sources that claim several immunosuppressant or immunostimulatory properties. The most common supplements reported by patients with rheumatic diseases are fish oil or omega-3 polyunsaturated fatty acids, gamma-linolenic acid and antioxidants (e.g. C, E and selenium). The scientific evidence so far does not justify the systematic use of such supplements, since some of them may exhibit serious side effects or interactions with the recommended medication. The most evidence-based information exists for the use of fish oils as part of the treatment for inflammatory disorders such as RA; however, the recommended effective doses remain a controversial issue. Antioxidant supplementation, while seeming to have plausibility, lacks a comparable evidence base and the only dietary supplements that doctors routinely recommend to most patients with rheumatic diseases are calcium and vitamin D.

Further reading

Avenell A, Handoll HH (2006) Nutritional supplementation for hip fracture aftercare in older people. Cochrane Database of Systematic Reviews 2010, Issue 1. Art. No.: CD001880. DOI: 10.1002/14651858.CD001880.pub5.

Cashman KD (2007) Diet, nutrition, and bone health. Journal of Nutrition 137(suppl. 11): S2507–12.

Choi HK (2005) Dietary risk factors for rheumatic diseases. Current Opinion in Rheumatology 17(2): 141–6.

Choi HK, Atkinson K, Karlson EW et al. (2004) Purine-rich foods, dairy and protein intake, and the risk of gout in men. New England Journal of Medicine 350(11): 1093–103.

Goulding (2002) Major minerals: Calcium and magnesium. In: Essentials of Human Nutrition, (eds J Mann, AS Truswell). Oxford University Press, Oxford, pp. 129–43.

Heaney RP (2006) Absorbability and utility of calcium in mineral waters. American Journal of Clinical Nutrition 84(2): 371–4.

Holick MF (2002) Vitamin D: The underappreciated D-lightful hormone that is important for skeletal and cellular health. Current Opinion in Endocrinology and Diabetes 9(1): 87–98.

Holick MF (2005) The influence of vitamin D on bone health across the life cycle. Journal of Nutrition 135(11): S2726–7.

Key TJ, Appleby PN, Rosell MS (2006) Health effects of vegetarian and vegan diets. Proceedings of the Nutrition Society 65(1): 35–41.

Ortiz Z, Shea B, Suarez AM et al. (1999) Folic acid and folinic acid for reducing side effects in patients receiving methotrexate for rheumatoid arthritis. Cochrane Database of Systematic Reviews 1999, Issue 4. Art. No.: CD000951. DOI: 10.1002/14651858.CD000951.

Rall LC, Roubenoff R (2004) Rheumatoid cachexia: Metabolic abnormalities, mechanisms and interventions. Rheumatology (Oxford) 43(10): 1219–23.

Rennie KL, Hughes J, Lang R, Jebb SA (2003) Nutritional management of rheumatoid arthritis: A review of the evidence. Journal of Human Nutrition and Dietetics 16(2): 97–109.

Schlesinger N (2005) Dietary factors and hyperuricaemia. Current Pharmaceutical Design 11(32): 4133–8.

Shapses SA, Riedt CS (2006) Bone, body weight, and weight reduction: What are the concerns? *Journal of Nutrition* **136**(6): 1453–6.

Stamp LK, James MJ, Cleland LG (2005) Diet and rheumatoid arthritis: A review of the literature. *Seminars in Arthritis and Rheumatism* **35**(2): 77–94.

Stratton RJ, Ek AC, Engfer M *et al.* (2005) Enteral nutritional support in prevention and treatment of pressure ulcers: A systematic review and meta-analysis. *Ageing Research Reviews* **4**(3): 422–50.

Walsmith J, Roubenoff R (2002) Cachexia in rheumatoid arthritis. *International Journal of Cardiology* **85**(1): 89–99.

Weaver CM, Plawecki KL (1994). Dietary calcium: Adequacy of a vegetarian diet. *American Journal of Clinical Nutrition* **59**(suppl. 5): S1238–41.

Zhao LJ, Jiang H, Papasian CJ *et al.* (2008) Correlation of obesity and osteoporosis: Effect of fat mass on the determination of osteoporosis. *Journal of Bone and Mineral Research* **23**(1): 17–29.

Chapter 15
Nutrition and Anaemias

Kalliopi-Anna Poulia

What are the main causes of iron-deficiency anaemia? Who is most vulnerable to iron deficiency?

Iron-deficiency anaemia is a condition characterised by inadequate iron deposits in the body. Iron deficiency is the commonest nutritional deficiency and it occurs when body iron stores are insufficient to support the necessary rate of red blood cell production and haem synthesis in the bone marrow, to maintain a normal circulating red cell mass and haemoglobin concentration.

It can be caused by an inadequate dietary daily intake, increased demands due to pregnancy or growth and/or by increased blood losses (menstrual losses, haemorrhage or trauma).

The main symptoms of iron deficiency include fatigue, shortness of breath and vertigo.

Periods of life with increased vulnerability of iron-deficiency anaemia include adolescence (particularly among girls after the onset of menstruation), women during pregnancy or of childbearing age, infants and older people.

What are the main laboratory tests to evaluate iron-deficiency anaemia and iron status in the body?

Haemoglobin and serum ferritin are the most common ways to detect anaemia. The World Health Organization (WHO) criteria for the detection of anaemia, established in 1975, are the most widely accepted. Haemoglobin concentrations below 13 g/dl for adult males, 12 g/dl for menstruating women and 11 g/dl in pregnancy are considered indicative of anaemia. The main laboratory tests used for the detection of iron-deficiency anaemia are summarised in Table 15.1.

Table 15.1 Laboratory evaluation of iron-deficiency anaemia.

Aim of the test	Laboratory test
Confirm the presence of anaemia	Haemoglobin
	Haematocrit
Evaluate iron status	
Iron stores	Bone marrow iron
	Serum ferritin
Iron supply	Serum transferrin receptor concentration
	Transferrin saturation
	Free erythrocyte protoporphyrin
	Red blood cells indices
	Serum iron

What are the main dietary sources of iron?

There are two types of iron in the diet:

- Haem iron derived from haemoglobin and myoglobin, which represents a small fraction of total iron in the diet and is highly absorbed. Haem iron is provided by animal-origin foods (i.e. red meat and meat products, liver, kidneys, egg yolk, fish, chicken, etc.).
- Non-haem iron, which is inorganic iron, very abundant in vegetable foods and in fortified foods (i.e. dried fruits and vegetables, wholegrain cereals, legumes and fortified bread and cereals).

The bioavailability of non-haem iron is much lower than haem iron and it depends on several dietary and physiological factors. The absorption of haem iron can range from 8 to 40%, while non-haem iron is absorbed by 0.5–6%. The average iron content of a typical Western diet is about 10–15 mg, of which only 10–15% is absorbed.

What factors interfere with iron absorption? What dietary factors play a role in iron bioavailability?

Haem iron, principally provided by meat, fish and blood-derived foods, as mentioned before, is better absorbed than non-haem iron is. Haem iron absorption can be altered only by meat presence and to a smaller degree by the presence of calcium. Haem iron absorption is higher in the presence of meat, by a mechanism still under investigation. Moreover, as meat is the best dietary source of iron, it enhances its absorption and significantly increases the dietary content of iron. It should also be stressed that heat treatment and storage can transform haem iron into non-haem iron, resulting in the lower absorption of iron from certain foods.

Table 15.2 Factors enhancing or inhibiting iron absorption.

Factors that enhance iron absorption	Factors that inhibit iron absorption
Haem iron	Non-haem iron
Acids (HCl, vitamin C)	Anti-acids
Amino acids, carbohydrates	Phytic and phosphate acids
Iron-deficiency anaemia	Tea, coffee
Pregnancy	Iron overload
Infancy	Infections
Adolescence	Gastrectomy
Hereditary haemochromatosis	Low levels of gastric acids

With respect to calcium, some studies have shown that calcium chloride inhibits haem iron absorption in the same extension as non-haem iron. Calcium seems to have a direct effect on haem iron absorption, counteracting the enhancing effect of meat. It has also been demonstrated that this inhibitory effect is dose-related, as a dose below 40 mg does not have an inhibitory effect, while maximum inhibition is reached with intakes around 300 mg, where the inhibition of iron absorption is almost complete.

The availability of non-haem iron further depends on dietetic factors and is generally considered lower. Its absorption is inhibited by the presence of phytic acid and polyphenols. According to recent scientific data, phenolic compounds found in spices and herbs (i.e. chilli, garlic, pepper, shallot and turmeric) are potent inhibitors of iron availability, reducing iron availability from 20 to 90% in a dose-dependent manner. Conversely, caseinophosphopeptides seem to improve iron absorption and availability either by increasing its solubility or by diminishing other interactions with other minerals. Moreover, vitamins like vitamin A and C enhance iron availability, thus counteracting the action of polyphenols and phytic acid.

Other factors that could enhance or inhibit iron absorption are summarised in Table 15.2.

What are the main components of the dietary advice that should be given to patients with iron-deficiency anaemia?

The aim of dietary advice in patients with iron-deficiency anaemia is to enhance the iron absorption of their food and to restore iron stores in the body. Patients should be advised to:

- include food items with high iron content in their daily diet
- consume sources of vitamin C in every meal, to enhance iron absorption
- consume food items with haem iron in every meal if possible
- avoid the consumption of large amounts of tea and coffee, especially with meals, as they could inhibit iron absorption
- consume up to three cups of milk or yogurt per day, as generally advised, but not with items rich in iron.

Chapter 15

What is haemochromatosis? What are the main symptoms and what is the dietary management of iron overload?

Haemochromatosis is an inherited or secondary condition that alters iron metabolism. It is the most common form of iron overload due to excessive iron absorption from the intestine. Physiologically, the only available mechanism in humans to prevent iron overload is the regulation of iron absorption in the intestine. Hereditary haemochromatosis is caused by a defect in a gene called HFE, which interferes with the regulation of dietary iron absorption from the small intestine. Haemochromatosis can also be due to repeated blood transfusions, African iron overload (previously known as African siderosis) and anaemia due to insufficient erythropoiesis, thalassaemia or Mediterranean anaemia.

Iron cannot be excreted and it can be toxic if it is accumulated in the human body. Even though haemochromatosis may be asymptomatic, it can be accompanied by symptoms such as chronic fatigue, abdominal pain, irregular heart rhythm, hair loss and changes in skin colour – not attributed to sun exposure. Haemochromatosis can cause serious health problems, mainly owing to iron accumulation in the organs, i.e. hepatic disorders (cirrhosis, hepatoma – with or without alcohol use), arthritis, gallstones, diabetes and heart disorders (heart failure, heart attack). It can be diagnosed by the measurement of elevated transferrin saturation (>50% for women and >60% for men), elevated ferritin levels and genetic tests to certify HFE gene mutations.

The main therapy for haemochromatosis is iron removal, either by blood donation (phlebotomy) or by pharmacological removal by chelation therapy. Dietary advice consists of ways to impair iron absorption from foods. Increasing fibre intake, avoiding the intake of vitamin C at mealtimes and the increased intake of dietary items with either low iron content or of low iron bioavailability is often recommended. Vitamin C and iron supplements should be avoided in these patients. Moreover, alcohol intake should be restricted as it can worsen the hepatic damage.

What are the main causes of megaloblastic anaemia?

Megaloblastic anaemia is characterised by the formation of abnormally large erythrocytes in the bone marrow and by abnormally large (macrocytic) erythrocytes and hyper-segmented neutrophils in the blood. Megaloblastic anaemia is caused by a reduction in the rate of DNA biosynthesis, resulting in abnormal nuclear maturation and ineffective erythropoiesis. The most common aetiology for megaloblastic anaemia is folate and B_{12} deficiencies. Other less common factors are the use of drugs that interrupt DNA biosynthesis and inherited conditions presenting defective enzymes of DNA biosynthesis.

What factors can cause B_{12} and folic-acid deficiency and what is the dietary management of these deficiencies?

In Western countries, B_{12} deficiency is mainly caused by pernicious anaemia. Pernicious anaemia is characterised by the insufficient production of the

Table 15.3 Causes of B$_{12}$ deficiency.

Malabsorption	Insufficient dietary intake

Stomach
    pernicious anaemia
    gastrectomy
	Vegetarianism

Bowel
    coeliac disease
    Crohn's disease
    ileoectomy
    infection by fish tapeworm
    diverticulum
    fistulas	

intrinsic factor in the stomach, which is essential for the absorption of B$_{12}$. Other less common causes include vegetarianism, gastrectomy and bowel disorders (Table 15.3).

The dietary management of B$_{12}$ deficiency includes a high-protein diet (1.5 g/kg body weight), a higher consumption of green leafy vegetables and inclusion of food items rich in B$_{12}$, i.e. meat, eggs and dairy products.

Folic acid deficiency is usually a result of a diet low in this vitamin, in combination with lower absorption and/or higher needs (Table 15.4). Pregnancy is characterised by an increased need of folic acid, while medication for epilepsy and barbiturates can cause folate deficiency. Moreover, alcohol consumption can alter folate metabolism and absorption.

Foods with a high folate content include green leafy vegetables, fruits, breakfast cereals and dairy products. Folate is sensitive to high temperatures, and cooking can destroy 50–95% of folate in the foods. Therefore, patients should be advised to consume fresh fruit and vegetables in order to increase their dietary intake of this vitamin.

Table 15.4 Causes of folate deficiency.

Insufficient dietary intake	Malabsorption	Increased needs	Increased urinary losses	Medications
	coeliac disease Crohn's disease	pregnancy, premature infants, lactation haemolytic anaemia cancer, lymphomas inflammatory diseases (psoriasis, rheumatoid arthritis)	hepatic disease heart disease	antiepileptic barbiturates

Chapter 15

Further reading

Amaro López MA, Camara Martos F (2004) Iron availability: An updated review. *International Journal of Food Sciences and Nutrition* **55**(8): 597–606.

Bendich A (2001) Calcium supplementation and iron status of females. *Nutrition* **17**(1): 46–51.

Centers for Disease Control (1998) Recommendations to prevent and control iron deficiency in the United States. *Morbidity and Mortality Weekly Report* **47**: 1–29.

Cook JD (2005) Diagnosis and management of iron-deficiency anaemia. *Best Practice & Research Clinical Haematology* **18**(2): 319–32.

Fowler C (2008) Hereditary hemochromatosis: Pathophysiology, diagnosis, and management. *Critical Care Nursing Clinics of North America* **20**(2): 191–201.

Gräsbeck R (2005) Megaloblastic anaemia (MA). *Hematology* **10**: 227–8.

Hercberg S, Preziosi P, Galan P (2001) Iron deficiency in Europe. *Public Health Nutrition* **4**(2B): 537–45.

Tuntipopipat S, Zeder C, Siriprapa P, Charoenkiatkul S (2008) Inhibitory effects of spices and herbs on iron availability. *International Journal of Food Sciences and Nutrition* **24**: 1–13.

Zimmermann MB, Hurrell RF (2007) Nutritional iron deficiency. *Lancet* **370**(9586): 511–20.

Chapter 16

Neurological and Mental Disorders

Kalliopi-Anna Poulia

What are the main signs and symptoms of dysphagia?

Dysphagia, or difficulty in swallowing, is a common problem in patients with neurological diseases, often resulting in aspiration pneumonia, compromised nutrient intake, dehydration and malnutrition.

The main signs and symptoms of dysphagia include:

- excessive saliva excretion, choking and coughing during or after meals
- poor control of tongue, excessive tongue movement and spitting food out of the mouth
- inability to drink liquids through a straw
- pocketing of food in cheek or under tongue
- wet 'gurly' voice after eating or frequent throat clearing
- delayed or absent laryngeal elevation
- prolonged chewing or eating time
- chronic or recurrent upper respiratory problems.

What are the main nutritional goals for the treatment of a dysphagic patient?

The main goals for the nutritional management of a dysphagic patient are:

- the determination of the safest route for the provision of food, to prevent aspiration and choking.
- the evaluation of the problem and the assessment of the texture of the foods that the patient can tolerate.
- the provision of sufficient energy and nutrient intake, to ensure the best possible nutritional status of the patient.
- the intake of sufficient liquid to prevent dehydration.

Table 16.1 Description of food and fluid consistencies.

Consistency	Description
Foods	
Puréed	Pudding-like consistency, thick, homogenous textures
Ground or minced	Easily mashed foods, no coarse textures, raw fruits or vegetables (except for raw banana)
Soft or easy to chew	Soft foods prepared without use of blender; meats minced or cut in small pieces, no tough skins, nuts or raw crispy or stingy foods
Modified, general	Soft textures prepared without grinding or chopping; no nuts or crispy foods
Fluids	
Thin	Regular fluids
Nectar-like	Fluids thin enough to be sipped through a straw or a cup, but thick enough to fall off a tipped spoon slowly (e.g. buttermilk, milkshake)
Honey-like	Thick fluids eaten with a spoon, too thick for a straw and unable to hold their shape (e.g. thick yogurt, honey)
Spoon-thick	Pudding-like fluids that must be eaten with a spoon, that can hold their shape on a spoon (e.g. milk pudding, jelly)

What are the characteristics of the dietary regimens for patients with dysphagia?

Dysphagia diets must be highly individualised, depending on the patient's chewing and swallowing ability. Foods' texture and viscosity may be altered in order to be tolerated. Fluids and liquids are categorised in four groups, progressing form the easiest to most difficult to swallow. The description of food and fluid consistencies is included in Table 16.1.

What are the main problems caused by the texture and density manipulation of foods for dysphagic patients?

Food items used in puréed preparations should be thoroughly cooked. This causes the loss of a significant amount of their vitamin and mineral content and often the prescription of a multivitamin is necessary in order to ensure that the patient receives sufficient micronutrient intake. Moreover, constipation is very common among these patients, since texture manipulation through stirring and diluting the food items results in feeds relatively low in dietary fibre. Another problem that can also compromise the nutritional intake of dysphagic patients is the alteration in food appearance and smell following texture manipulation. The use of special equipment that can give special forms to the food and taste enhancers can be used in order to ensure food palatability and better patient compliance.

What are the aetiology and main clinical symptoms of pernicious anaemia? What is its nutritional management?

Pernicious anaemia was first described in 1948. It is a macrocytic, megaloblastic anaemia, caused by B_{12} deficiency or by secondary vitamin deficiency due to a lack in the intrinsic factor, which is excreted in the stomach and is necessary for the absorption of B_{12}. The overt symptoms of pernicious anaemia include paraesthesia, numbness and tingling of feet and hands, poor muscular coordination, poor memory and diminution of the sensation of vibration and position. Its treatment consists of intramuscular or subcutaneous injections of B_{12}. For the nutritional management of pernicious anaemia, food items such as meat, eggs and dairy foods are considered rich sources of vitamin B_{12} and should be included in the diet plan of the patient to ensure the sufficient dietary intake of this vitamin.

What are the main nutritional neuropathies? How are they treated?

Nutritional neuropathies mainly affect the peripheral nervous system, and their symptoms include lean body mass depletion and progressive wasting. Early signs are anorexia, irritability, weight loss and abdominal discomfort, while in the long term paralysis, numbness and the disturbance of a patient's sense of hot and cold may be observed. The most common forms of nutritional neuropathies – beriberi and alcoholic neuropathy – can be attributed to thiamin deficiency, but other deficiencies in B-complex vitamins cannot be excluded. The nutritional management of these neuropathies is a balanced diet with supplementation of B-complex vitamins. Specifically in alcoholic neuropathy, thiamin supplements should be added, and abstinence from alcohol is essential for the recovery of the patient.

Chapter 16

What are the nutritional needs of patients with a recent stroke? How may that stroke influence their nutritional status and their ability to feed themselves?

When a patient with a recent stroke is being evaluated, it must be taken into account that:

- A brain injury due to a stroke results in a hypercatabolic state for patients, raising their energy and protein needs significantly. Moreover, as insulin resistance and electrolyte imbalances are rather common in these patients, they should also be co-estimated.
- A stroke can severely modify the ability of the patient to receive food without help. Table 16.2 summarises the possible effects of the neurological disturbances caused by a stroke on the nutritional intake of the patient.

Table 16.2 Possible neurological consequences of stroke on nutritional intake.

Neurological deficit	Influence on nutritional parameters
Perception	Disturbed perception of time. Unable to identify meal times
Visual perception/ hemianopsia	Cannot define or recognise food items. In some cases only half of the plate is seen and therefore only half of the food is eaten
Spatial deficits	Unable to analyse position of the plate
Behaviour	Food thrown around and not eaten
Apraxia	Unable to use cutlery and self-feed
Aphasia	Forget to eat
Memory	Forget that he/she has already eaten
Hemiplegia	Able to use only one hand to self-feed
Ataxia	Unable to self-feed
Psychological influences/ depression	Limited appetite

- Malnutrition is common in patients with stroke, caused either by their increased nutritional needs or by their compromised nutritional intake, and can prolong the recovery or increase comorbidities, such as pressure ulcers and infections.

What is the role of diet in the cognitive decline of the older population?

Cognitive decline and dementia deeply affect the quality of life of older people and their caregivers. Therapeutic options for the treatment of Alzheimer's disease and dementia have been shown to be of limited efficacy, and prevention strategies are mandatory. There is cumulative evidence of the possible protective role of lifestyle and diet-related factors for the prevention of cognitive decline. At present, in older subjects, balanced diets, the prevention of nutritional deficiencies of antioxidants by nutritional supplements and moderate physical activity could be considered the first line of defence against the onset or progression of dementia. Moderate alcohol consumption seems to be a protective factor against mild cognitive impairment, dementia and Alzheimer's disease. Apart from alcohol, dietary models based on complex carbohydrates, fruits and vegetables and low in animal fat appear to protect against cognitive decline that is degenerative or vascular in origin, owing mainly to the high provision of antioxidants. Fish consumption has been associated with the lower risk of Alzheimer's disease in longitudinal cohort studies. Moreover, epidemiological data suggest a protective role of the B vitamins, especially vitamins B_9 and B_{12}, on cognitive decline and dementia. Moreover, the higher consumption of polyunsaturated and monounsaturated fatty acids seems to have a significant protective effect. The Mediterranean diet could therefore be an interesting model to investigate the possible role of specific dietary patterns and cognitive decline.

Conversely, vitamin deficiencies could have a negative impact on cognition in older people, while the aluminium content of foods and water may also affect the risk of developing Alzheimer's disease.

What is the ketogenic diet and what is its role in the treatment of epilepsy?

Ketogenic diets were first tested for the treatment of epilepsy in 1928. Nowadays, they are used for the treatment of akinetic, myoclonic, petit mal or psychomotor seizures in children, when they cannot be controlled by medication alone. These types of diets are designed to create and maintain a state of ketosis and their beneficial effect may be attributed to the role of ketone bodies as inhibitory neurotransmitters, providing an anticonvulsant effect to the patient.

There are two forms of ketogenic diets: the traditional one and the ketogenic diet based on medium-chain triglycerides (MCT). Both forms of these diets are calculated to provide 75% of the recommended dietary allowance (RDA) of energy for the child's ideal weight and height and a 4:1 ratio of kcal from fat to kcal from protein and carbohydrates respectively. But it must be borne in mind that the child receives sufficient protein provision to ensure growth (approximately 1 g/kg body weight/day). Fluids are controlled (approximately 65 ml/kg/day) and should not exceed 2 l/day.

The MCT approach provides 50–70% of kcals in the form of MCT oil. In the MCT approach, a greater amount of non-ketogenic food is allowed as ketosis can be more easily achieved with MCT oil, and fluid restriction is not necessary.

It should be stressed that the ketogenic diet is a difficult diet to follow, and can be nutritionally incomplete. Therefore, a multivitamin supplement is often needed to ensure the sufficient nutritional intake and growth of the child. Ketogenic diets are often discontinued after 2–3 years.

What nutritional problems are connected with multiple sclerosis?

One of the main problems associated with multiple sclerosis is malnutrition due to the loss of interest in, or inadequate consumption of, food. The aetiology of malnutrition in these patients is:

- psychological factors, e.g. anorexia or depression, as a result of the diagnosis
- side effects of the medical treatment
- fatigue and disability in preparing meals.

Apart from undernourishment, overweight and obesity due to limited physical exercise and increased appetite mainly due to corticosteroid therapy can also be observed in this population. Moreover, binge eating and bulimic episodes can be seen as a result of depression in these patients.

Chapter 16

It is also noteworthy that constipation is a common symptom, resulting from reduced mobility and physical exercise, restricted fluid intake due to problems in micturition or continence and reduced bowel movement due to the disease.

How can Parkinson's disease influence the nutritional status of the patient?

Parkinson's disease frequently affects patients' nutritional intake. The symptoms of the disease can vary between patients and may worsen as the disease progresses. They can include:

- tremor and rigidity, causing difficulties in preparing food and self-feeding
- slow movement, resulting in extended meal duration
- depression, limited appetite, apathy
- drug side effects (nausea, vomiting, anorexia)
- swallowing difficulties (dysphagia).

Patients with Parkinson's disease may also have increased energy requirements due to tremor and rigidity thus worsening the effects of an already inadequate intake.

What are the main nutritional interventions that can help patients with Parkinson's disease?

Nutritional intervention should aim to promote an adequate dietary intake, taking into account any difficulties in feeding due to symptoms of Parkinson's disease. Such interventions may include nutritional support (e.g. supplementation, tube feeding during the end stages of the disease and texture modification due to dysphagia). Table 16.3 proposes specific solutions for the problems that are usually seen in patients with Parkinson's disease.

How can the prescription of levodopa alter the design of a dietary plan for a patient with Parkinson's disease?

Levodopa (or L-DOPA) is used in the treatment of Parkinson's and has been found to be affected by dietary intake, particularly that of neutral amino acids, which compete with the levodopa and reduce its action. Recent interest has focused on the use of protein redistribution diets to optimise the action of Levodopa. This may involve limiting protein or redistributing it within the diet to reduce the protein load at breakfast and lunch and moving it to the evening meal. Interest has also arisen around the effects of antioxidant nutrients in the prevention of Parkinson's; however, there is no evidence to suggest that they have any effect on the progression of the disease.

Chapter 16

Table 16.3 Suggested actions for common problems of a patient with Parkinson's disease.

Problem	Action
Inadequate intake/ underweight	Food fortification (e.g. adding high-calorie products such as sugar, butter and cheese to appropriate foods, milk powder/cream to milk products/soups) Nutrient-dense foods (e.g. milk and dairy products, meat) Dietary supplementation (e.g. prescribable or non-prescribable sip feeds)
Swallowing difficulties	Texture modification, under advice of speech and language therapist
Tremor	Large-handled cutlery, two-handled cup, non-slip mat/damp cloth under plate (liaise with occupational therapist)
Drug side effects	Dietary modification to reduce nausea and vomiting (e.g. dry foods, exclusion of trigger foods)
Constipation	Increase fibre (e.g. increase fruit and vegetables, high-fibre options, such as wholemeal bread, bran/fibre cereals) and fluid
Overweight	Advice on diet through dietitian, and exercise (liaise with physiotherapist)

What are the most common nutritional implications of mood disorders?

The main types of mood disorders are depression, anxiety and mania. Its nutritional implications depend on the severity of the disorder, and some of the most common ones are summarised in Table 16.4. Severe depression can alter a patient's interest in food, either by increasing the amount of food consumed or by causing anorexia or food refusal. Moreover, mainly owing to neurotransmitter imbalance, depression can cause carbohydrate cravings, resulting in weight gain. Depression can also diminish thirst sensation, resulting in a high risk of dehydration for these patients.

Table 16.4 Common implications of mood disorders.

Mood disorder	Influence on food intake	Nutritional implication
Depression	Reduced interest in food, apathy, anorexia, food refusal	Weight loss, malnutrition
	Loss of thirst sensation	Dehydration, constipation
	Carbohydrate cravings	Weight gain, dietary imbalances
Anxiety	Diarrhoea, abdominal pain or discomfort	Selective avoidance of food groups, excessive nutrient losses
Mania	Xerostomia and altered taste due to drugs' side effects	Difficulties in chewing and swallowing
	Increased appetite	Weight gain, obesity
	Strange food habits	Nutrient imbalances, weight gain

Chapter 16

Anxiety can also have an effect on the nutritional status of the patient. It is often accompanied by diarrhoea and abdominal pain or discomfort, causing the selective avoidance of food groups and excessive nutrient losses.

Finally, mania can be accompanied by unusual eating habits and increased appetite, causing weight gain and nutritional imbalance. Moreover, drug side effects include taste alterations and xerostomia, resulting in difficulties in swallowing and chewing.

What precautions should be taken for patients receiving treatment with lithium?

Lithium salts are used for the treatment of mania and have a very narrow range between therapeutic effectiveness and toxicity. Therefore, they should be used only for the period they are necessary, as their long-term use is connected with undesired effects on renal function. Moreover, there is an inverse relationship between sodium intake and serum lithium levels, and toxicity from lithium can be a result of sodium restriction. Patients receiving therapy with lithium should be encouraged to maintain sufficient fluid intake and avoid dietary modifications that could alter their sodium intake.

What are the main causes of obesity in patients with mental illnesses?

Obesity in mentally ill patients is a common problem. It can be attributed mainly to the side effects of their medications (i.e. increased appetite, carbohydrate cravings, direct effects on metabolic, endocrinological and neurochemical mechanisms) but can be the result of other reasons as well. Reduced physical activity and disturbed judgement on food choice, along with poor nutritional knowledge, can cause weight gain in these patients. The common belief that antidepressant and antipsychotic drugs can cause weight gain is often a reason for poor medication compliance. Therefore, coordination between therapists and dietitians may be very useful in order to avoid excessive weight gain and assure compliance with drug regimens.

Further reading

Carter JH, Nutt JG, Woodward WR et al. (1989) Amount and distribution of dietary protein affects clinical response to levodopa in Parkinson's disease. *Neurology* **39**: 552–6.

Gillette Guyonnet Abellan S, Van Kan G, Andrieu S et al. (2007) IANA task force on nutrition and cognitive decline with aging. *Journal of Nutrition, Health & Aging* **11**(2): 132–52.

Chapter 16

Kempster PA, Wahlqvist ML (1994) Dietary factors in the management of Parkinson's disease. *Nutrition Reviews* **52**(2, part 2): 51–8.

Kumar N (2007) Nutritional neuropathies. *Neurologic Clinics.* **25**(1): 209–55.

Lakhan SE, Vieira KF (2008) Nutritional therapies for mental disorders. *Nutrition Journal* **7**: 2.

Levy R, Cooper P (2003) Ketogenic diet for epilepsy. Cochrane Database of Systematic Reviews 2003, Issue 3. Art. No.: CD001903. DOI: 10.1002/14651858.CD001903.

Riley D, Land AE (1998) Practical application of low protein diet for Parkinson disease. *Neurology* **38**: 1026–31.

Solfrizzi V, Panza F, Capurso A (2003) The role of diet in cognitive decline. *Journal of Neural Transmission* **110**(1): 95–110.

Strowd L, Kyzima J, Pillsbury D *et al.* (2008) Dysphagia dietary guidelines and the rheology of nutritional feeds and barium test feeds. *Chest* **133**(6): 1397–401.

Timmerman GM, Stuifbergin AK (1999) Eating patterns in women with multiple sclerosis. *Journal of Neuroscience Nursing* **31**(3): 152–8.

Thomas B (2007) *Manual of Dietetic Practice*, (3rd edn). Blackwell Science Ltd, Oxford.

Chapter 16

Chapter 17

Enteral Nutrition

Kalliopi-Anna Poulia

What are the types of enteral nutrition? What specifies the decision for the type of nutritional support given to a patient?

The two main categories of enteral nutrition are enteral tube feeding and oral nutritional supplements. Before deciding to provide nutritional support to a patient enterally, it is important to take into account:

- the predicted duration of the provision of the nutritional support
- the danger of aspiration or tube misplacement
- the presence or absence of digestion and absorption, i.e. the level of gastrointestinal (GI) functionality
- whether a surgical operation is programmed
- the texture and the volume of the feed that should be provided in order to meet the patient's needs.

What is enteral tube feeding and when should it be administered? What are the routes of its administration?

Enteral tube feeding (ETF) is the provision of nutrients by a tube through the GI tract in patients who cannot attain sufficient oral intake from food and/or oral nutritional supplements or who cannot nourish themselves safely for periods of more than five days (e.g. dysphagic patients). It aims to maintain a patient's nutritional status and to improve their nutritional intake. ETF should be administered in patients with an accessible and functional GI tract – a minimum of 100 cm of functional jejunum, a minimum of 150 cm of functional ileum and some colon, preferably with an intact ileocecal valve – to ensure the sufficient digestion and absorption of the feed. The common indications for the provision of ETF are summarised in Table 17.1. If ETF is unsafe or unsuccessful, other routes of artificial support should be chosen (i.e. parenteral nutrition; see Chapter 18).

Table 17.1 Indications for the provision of enteral tube feeding.

Indication	Clinical example
Unconscious patient	Head injury, mechanical ventilation, stroke, ICU patients
Anorexia	Neoplasm, liver disease, HIV, depression, anorexia nervosa
Upper-GI obstruction	Oropharyngeal or oesophageal stricture or tumour
GI dysfunction	Inflammatory bowel disease
Malabsorption	Short bowel syndrome
Mental illness	Alzheimer's disease, dementia
Increased requirements	Burns, cystic fibrosis

The route of ETF is decided on an individual basis, according to the patient's clinical condition and nutritional status, the treatment followed and the predicted duration of the nourishment by ETF. ETF can be delivered:

- directly to the stomach (gastric feeding) via:
    - a nasogastric tube: usually used for short-term feeding (<14 days)
    - gastrostomy or percutaneus endoscopic gastrostomy (PEG), commonly used for long-term ETF
    - oesophagostomy, less common
- beyond the stomach via:
    - a nasoduodenal or nasojejunal tube, in cases where the stomach has to be bypassed, lower risk of aspiration
    - gastrojejunostomy, usually in patients with pre-existing gastrostomy
    - jejunostomy, usually in patients who have undergone major GI or hepatobiliary operations, or in cases of increased risk of gastric paresis.

What are oral supplements and when should they be used?

Oral supplements are usually pre-packed drinks, pills or powder-like substances, with a significant nutrient content, prescribed to improve the nutritional status of patients who fail to meet their nutritional requirements through food intake alone. Oral nutritional supplements can be categorised as follows:

- Complete oral supplements, which contain macro- and micronutrients. Usually they are prescribed as a supplement to the daily intake of foods, but the majority of them can be provided as exclusive nutrition. The content of these feeds in macronutrients varies and there are supplements for general use or for specific clinical conditions.
- Oral supplements with modified nutrient content, i.e. hydrolysed or partially hydrolysed, elemental or semi-elemental feeds, fat-free, etc.

Table 17.2 Classification of enteral feeds.

Type of feed	Description
General feeds (polymeric)	For patients with normal digestion and absorption. They contain whole proteins. Usual osmolarity: 300–500 mOsm/kg, 1–1.2 kcal/ml, 30–40 g protein/l
Hydrolysed/elemental	For patients with limited GI function. They contain free amino acids, low in fat and low residue. Hyperosmotic, 1 kcal/ml, 40 g protein/L. Expensive
Semi-elemental/ partially hydrolysed/ peptide feeds	For patients with disturbed GI function, who need partially hydrolysed nutrients for better digestion and absorption. Osmolarity: depends on the level of hydrolysis, 1–1.2 kcal/ml, 30–45 g protein/l. Relatively expensive
Disease-specific enteral formulae	Designed for specific clinical conditions and metabolic disorders (i.e. chronic renal failure, respiratory disease, diabetes, cancer). Expensive

- Supplements of one or more macronutrients, i.e. carbohydrate, fat or protein.
- Multivitamin supplements.

Oral nutritional support should be considered for malnourished patients or those in danger of insufficient nutrient intake through food, presupposing that they can swallow safely and they have an adequately functioning GI.

How are the types of enteral feeds classified?

Most enteral feeds are ready-to-use fluids, in microbial-free containers that provide macronutrients, micronutrients, fluids and, in some cases, soluble or insoluble fibre. They are usually nutritionally complete within a specific volume, providing the necessary nutrients to support the dietary needs of the patient.

Table 17.2 shows the classification of enteral feeds.

What are the indications for using elemental or semi-elemental enteral feeds?

Elemental and semi-elemental feeds facilitate digestion and absorption in patients with a problematic GI function. They are indicated for patients with inflammatory bowel disease, pancreatic insufficiency, malabsorption, short bowel syndrome, radiation enteritis, early enteral feeding or intolerance to polymeric feeds.

What are the main characteristics of renal, pulmonary, hepatic and diabetic feeds?

Renal feeds

They usually contain limited amounts of sodium, potassium and phosphorus. Their protein content varies: there are low-protein feeds for the early stages of chronic kidney disease (CKD) and higher-protein feeds for end-stage CKD patients (i.e. patients undergoing hemodialysis or peritoneal dialysis). The feeds for end-stage CKD patients are usually energy-dense, facilitating the fluid restriction that is needed for them.

Pulmonary feeds

They usually contain a higher percentage of their total energy in the form of fat to reduce the carbon dioxide that is produced by the feed metabolism.

Hepatic feeds

These are commonly low in aromatic amino acids (AAA) and methionine and high in branched-chain amino acids (BCAA). They usually have a high calorie/nitrogen ratio, are hypercaloric, low in sodium and contain dietary fibre to promote gut motility. They are usually low in copper, iron and manganese and are supplemented with fat-soluble vitamins, folic acid and B-complex vitamins.

Diabetic feeds

They usually have a lower carbohydrate content and a type of carbohydrate that is different from the standard formulas. They usually contain oligosaccharides, fructose and cornstarch, and in combination with their higher fibre content they aim at better glycaemic control as a result of delayed gastric emptying and a reduced intestinal transit.

What are the main characteristics of immunonutrition? When may it be useful?

The potential to modulate the activity of the immune system by interventions with specific nutrients is termed 'immunonutrition'. Immunonutrition has three targets: mucosal barrier function, cellular defence and local or systemic inflammation. The nutrients that have been proven to play a role in the regulation of the immune system are the amino acids glutamine and arginine, BCAA, omega-3 fatty acids, dietary nucleotides, fructo-oligosaccharides (FOS) and antioxidants. Immune feeds contain variable amounts of these nutrients and are more expensive than general feeds. Usually they are prescribed for critically ill patients, in septic conditions or post-surgically.

What types of fibre are found in enteral formulas and what is their role?

Enteral feeds with dietary fibre contain both soluble and insoluble fibre. Soluble fibres, such as guar, pectin and FOS, are used as prebiotics. These substances are fermented by the colonic bacteria and short-chain fatty acids (SFAs) are produced. SFAs provide energy to colonocytes, improve mucosal growth and improve water and sodium absorption. Insoluble fibre increases faecal volume, enteral peristalsis and thereby decreases faecal transit time.

Enteral feeds with dietary fibre are recommended for patients with long-term enteral nutrition as they promote mucosal growth and gut peristalsis.

What are the contraindications for the use of enteral nutrition?

The use of enteral nutrition presupposes a sufficient functionality of the GI tract. Therefore, its use is contraindicated in specific clinical conditions that are characterised by compromised GI functionality, i.e. complete intestinal obstruction, intractable vomiting, paralytic ileus, circulatory shock, GI haemorrhage, short bowel, severe diarrhoea, GI ischemia and high output (>500 ml/day) enterocutaneous fistula.

What parameters should be monitored in patients receiving enteral nutritional support?

Following the initiation of enteral nutritional support, frequent monitoring of the patient is essential, in order to ensure the early detection and treatment of possible complications, to check the tolerability of the feed and to make sure that the goals of the nutritional support are fulfilled. The main parameters that should be monitored are summarised in Table 17.3.

Table 17.3 Monitoring enteral nutrition.

Parameter	Frequency
Weight	At least three times/week
Signs of oedema	Daily
Signs of dehydration	Daily
Fluid balance	Daily
Adequacy of provided nutritional support	At least twice/week
Nitrogen balance	Weekly
Gastric residues	Every four hours
Electrolytes; blood, urine, nitrogen (BUN); creatinine	2–3 times/week
Blood glucose, Ca, Mg, P	Weekly
Frequency and consistency of defecation	Daily

Chapter 17

What are the main complications of enteral tube feeding and how should they be managed?

The main complications of ETF include:

- Gastric retention and aspiration. Delayed gastric emptying is the main cause for the regurgitation of stomach contents and aspiration. Aspiration into the lungs can cause death due to asphyxia, or if the amount of the feed is small it can increase the risk of pneumonia. In patients with a high risk of aspiration special measures should be taken. More specifically:
  - ○ the position of the tube should be regularly checked
  - ○ the head and the upper body should be elevated by at least 30 degrees during feeding and one hour following feeding
  - ○ gastric emptying can be stimulated by the use of specific agents
  - ○ other routes of ETF, preferably post-pyloric, should be considered.
- Diarrhoea is a common complication of patients fed with ETF. It can be caused by a higher-than-appropriate rate of the feed administration, prolonged use of antibiotics, which can cause pathological bacteria overgrowth in the gut, and by the use of high-osmolarity feeds. Measures to alleviate diarrhoea include:
  - ○ the gradual initiation of the infusion of the feed. If the rate of infusion is suspected to be high, it should be decreased. The use of an infusion pump to ensure a stable infusion rate is preferable to bolus or gravity feeding
  - ○ selection of a feed with lower osmolarity
  - ○ use of feeds with soluble dietary fibre, which act as prebiotics in the gut
  - ○ faecal sample analysis to exclude pathological bacterial overgrowth
  - ○ in cases of malabsorption, the selection of an elemental feed is needed.
- Constipation is mainly caused by the fact that standard feeds are usually low-residue, containing no or insignificant amounts of dietary fibre. Therefore, for constipation a feed with soluble and insoluble fibre should be chosen. Moreover, the fluid status of the patient should be evaluated.
- Tube blockage is more often in patients receiving puréed food items through the tube. It can also be caused by the use of tubes that have a very small diameter, insufficient flushing of the tube or by the infusion of drugs in the form of powder or crushed pills via the tube. In order to avoid this complication:
  - ○ the tube should be flushed regularly, when tube feeding is discontinued or when drugs are administered through the tube
  - ○ drugs should be administered in syrup form whenever possible rather than pills, even if they are thoroughly crushed.
- Stoma site complications such as leakage, exit-site infections, necrotising fasciitis and pneumoperitoneum. These complications can be minimised by the use of aseptic conditions during the preparation of the feed, regular

assessment of the stoma site and good personal hygiene of the patient and their carers.

What is refeeding syndrome and how can it be avoided?

Refeeding syndrome is a potentially fatal but often undiagnosed complication that occurs in severely malnourished patients due to any cause. The aggressive initiation of feeding after prolonged starvation may precipitate numerous metabolic and pathophysiological alterations, leading to severe cardiac, respiratory, hepatic, haematological and neuromuscular complications and even death.

Patients at particular risk of experiencing refeeding syndrome are patients with at least one of the following criteria:

- BMI $\leq 16\,kg/m^2$
- a recent unintentional weight loss of $>15\%$ of their usual body weight
- very limited nutritional intake for >10 days and/or a low plasma concentration of potassium, phosphorus or magnesium prior to the initiation of refeeding.

Furthermore, patients with two or more of the following are also at high risk of developing refeeding syndrome:

- BMI $<18.5\,kg/m^2$
- very limited nutritional intake for >5 days
- a history of alcohol abuse
- use of drugs including insulin, chemotherapy or diuretics.

It should be stressed that refeeding syndrome has no specific clinical features and therefore may easily go unrecognised. Its predominant biochemical sign is hypophoshataemia, while other features can be observed, such as rapid decreases of potassium, magnesium or sodium levels and water retention. These fluid and electrolyte abnormalities can lead to dehydration, cardiac or respiratory failure, rhabdomyolysis, seizures, coma, hypotension and sudden death.

In order to prevent refeeding syndrome in patients receiving artificial nutritional support, it is vital to closely monitor their fluid balance and electrolyte status. Patients at high risk of developing refeeding syndrome who need artificial nutritional support should be identified. In these patients, the initiation of feeding should be very gradual, with a reduced calorie rate of their estimated dietary requirements (approximately 20 kcal/kg/day) to prevent the development of refeeding syndrome. Moreover, measurements of electrolytes and biochemical parameters (creatinine, urea, potassium, magnesium, phosphorus) should be performed daily for at least four days after the initiation of the provision of enteral feeding.

Chapter 17

Further reading

ASPEN Board of Directors and Clinical Guidelines Task Force (2002) Guidelines for the use of parenteral and enteral nutrition in adult and pediatric patients. *Journal of Parenteral and Enteral Nutrition* **26**(suppl. 1): 1–137SA.

Calder PC (2003) Immunonutrition. *British Medical Journal* **327**(7407): 117–8.

DeLegge MH (2008) Enteral feeding. *Current Opinion in Gastroenterology* **24**(2): 184–9.

Gariballa S (2008) Refeeding syndrome: A potentially fatal condition but remains underdiagnosed and undertreated. *Nutrition* **24**(6): 604–6.

Grand MJ, Martin S (2000) Delivery of enteral nutrition. *AACN Clinical Issues* **11**(4): 507–16.

Jeejeebhoy KN (2005) Enteral feeding. *Current Opinion in Gastroenterology* **21**(2): 187–91.

Kirby DF (2001) Decisions for enteral access in the intensive care unit. *Nutrition* **17**(9): 776–9.

Kreymann KG, Berger MM, Deutz NEP *et al.* (2006) ESPEN Guidelines on Enteral Nutrition: Intensive care. *Clinical Nutrition* **25**(2): 210–23.

Lochs H, Allison SP, Meier R *et al.* (2006) Introductory to the ESPEN Guidelines on Enteral Nutrition: Terminology, definitions and general topics. *Clinical Nutrition* **25**(2): 180–5.

Luft VC, Beghetto MG, de Mello ED, Polanczyk CA (2008) Role of enteral nutrition in the incidence of diarrhea among hospitalized adult patients. *Nutrition* **24**(6): 528–35.

National Institute for Health and Clinical Excellence (2006) *Nutrition Support in Adults: Oral nutrition support, enteral tube feeding and parenteral nutrition (Clinical Guideline 32)*. NICE, London, http://www.nice.org.uk/nicemedia/pdf/cg032fullguideline.pdf.

Nisim AA, Allins AD (2005) Enteral nutrition support. *Nutrition* **21**(1): 109–12.

Rushdi TA, Pichard C, Khater YH (2004) Control of diarrhea by fiber-enriched diet in ICU patients on enteral nutrition: a prospective randomized controlled trial. *Clinical Nutrition* **23**(6): 1344–52.

Stanga Z, Brunner A, Leuenberger M *et al.* (2008) Nutrition in clinical practice: The refeeding syndrome: Illustrative cases and guidelines for prevention and treatment. *European Journal of Clinical Nutrition* **62**(6): 687–94.

Stratton RJ, Elia M (2007) A review of reviews: A new look at the evidence for oral nutritional supplements in clinical practice. *Clinical Nutrition Supplement* **2**: 5–23.

Thomas B (2007) *Manual of Dietetic Practice*, (3rd edn). Blackwell Science Ltd, Oxford.

Chapter 18

Parenteral Nutrition

Kalliopi-Anna Poulia

What is parenteral nutrition? When should it be initiated?

Parenteral nutrition (PN) is the intravenous provision of nutrients, without using the gastrointestinal (GI) system. It should be considered for patients with:

- malnutrition or inadequate or unsafe oral and/or enteral nutritional intake
- GI functionality insufficient to support an adequate degree of digestion and absorption of nutrients, due to ileus, dysmotility, fistulae, surgical resection, etc.
- prolonged GI system failure (>5 days) or intestinal failure which is predicted to last for >5 days.

PN may also be chosen in patients who cannot tolerate enteral feeding (EF) or when EF is unsafe or impractical.

What are the routes of parenteral nutritional administration?

PN can be provided via catheter in:

- A peripheral vein dedicated solely to PN. As peripheral veins cannot support the infusion of hypertonic parenteral solutions, peripheral parenteral nutrition (PPN) should be chosen for short-term nutritional support (<14 days), as it can only partially cover the patient's nutritional needs.
- A central vein with high blood flow, either by a dedicated centrally placed central venous catheter or by a free dedicated lumen in a multilumen centrally placed catheter. Central parenteral nutrition or total parenteral nutrition (TPN) should be provided through tunnelling subclavian lines for long-term use (>30 days), while other central veins can also be used (cephalic vein or internal jugular vein). For TPN of shorter duration, non-tunnelling lines can be used.

What are the differences between peripheral parenteral nutrition and total parenteral nutrition? What are the main candidates for receiving each type of parenteral nutrition?

PPN is the provision of nutrients through a peripheral vein. The parenteral solution should not exceed 800–900 mOsm/kg to prevent thrombophlebitis, the main complication of PPN. As peripheral veins cannot tolerate concentrated solutions, nutritional needs can be met with larger volumes of solutions, or can be covered only partially, especially if there is a fluid restriction for the patient (e.g. patients with renal, cardiopulmonary or hepatic failure). Therefore, PPN should be used for short-term parenteral nutritional support (<14 days), while it is also suggested that PPN should be used as a supplementary nutritional support or during the transitional phase from parenteral to enteral or oral feeding.

TPN is the provision of nutrients through a central vein. In TPN hypertonic solutions can be safely used, resulting in the provision of solutions with a higher calorie content but with lower volumes.

What should the monitoring of critically ill patients receiving PN include and how often should these values be obtained?

The provision of PN presupposes – just like the provision of enteral nutritional support – regular monitoring, in order to ensure the safety of the patient and the achievement of the goals of their nutritional support.

The suggested frequency of monitoring during PN is summarised in Table 18.1.

Table 18.1 Monitoring of parenteral nutritional support.

Parameter	Frequency
Temperature	Daily
Fluid balance	Daily
Blood and urine glucose	Every 6–8 hours
Electrolytes	Daily
Urea/creatinine	Daily
Calcium, phosphorus	Twice weekly
Liver function tests	Twice weekly
Albumin/total protein	Twice weekly
Cholesterol	Weekly
Nitrogen balance	Weekly
Magnesium	Weekly
Weight	Weekly

How can the nutritional needs of critically ill patients be calculated?

The assessment of a patient's nutritional needs is essential in order to ensure the sufficient provision of nutrients through nutritional support.

Energy

Usually, the energy needs of the patient can be estimated by the calculation of their basal metabolic rate, ideally by indirect calorimetry. Owing to the high cost of the equipment for indirect calorimetry, in the clinical setting the use of appropriate equations taking account of the age, sex, body weight and additional increments depending on the metabolic stress of the patients are a more common means of assessment. For the majority of patients, the provision of 20–30 kcal/kg seems to be adequate, while for severely malnourished patients or those at risk of refeeding syndrome lower levels of energy intake should be chosen.

Protein

Protein needs are estimated according to the body weight of the patient, with relevant variations due to metabolic stress or illness. Typically, the provision of 1.0 g/kg of protein (corresponding in 0.15 g nitrogen from amino acids) is sufficient for most patients. In situations of severe metabolic stress requirements could be higher (i.e. 1.0–1.5 g/kg), while in patients with renal or hepatic failure lower protein intakes are advised.

Fluids

Fluids should be about 30–35 ml/kg per day, adding possible fluid losses owing to drains fistulae, etc. All sources of fluids should be calculated to avoid the excessive provision of fluid.

Micronutrients and electrolytes

As the parenteral provision of micronutrients does not go through digestion and absorption, the recommended daily allowances are lower than those for oral nutrition. The majority of pre-prepared PN feeds contain variable amounts of electrolytes, while there are others which are electrolyte-free for patients with renal or hepatic failure. Regarding micronutrients, most feeds contain insignificant amounts of vitamins and minerals and therefore should be added to the feed. The recommended daily amounts of micronutrients for patients receiving PN are summarised in Table 18.2.

Chapter 18

Table 18.2 Recommended daily amounts of micronutrients for patients receiving parenteral nutrition.

Electrolytes	Parenteral equivalent of recommended daily amounts	Usual provision by the feeds
Ca	10 mEq	10–15 mEq
Mg	10 mEq	8–20 mEq
P	30 mmol	20–40 mmol
Na	N/A	1–2 mEq/kg + addition where needed
K	N/A	1–2 mEq/kg
Cl	N/A	As needed to maintain acid–base balance
Acetate	N/A	As needed to maintain acid–base balance
Vitamins		*Intake*
Thiamin (B$_1$)		3.0 mg
Riboflavin (B$_2$)		3.6 mg
Niacin (B$_3$)		40.0 mg
Folic acid		400.0 mg
Pantothenic acid		15.0 mg
B$_6$		4.0 mg
B$_{12}$		5.0 µg
Biotin		60.0 µg
C (ascorbic acid)		100.0 mg
A		3300.0 IU
D		200.0 IU
E		10.0 IU
Trace elements		*Intake*
Chromium		10–15 µg
Copper		0.3–0.5 mg
Manganese		60–100 µg
Zinc		2.5–5.0 mg

What is refeeding syndrome and how can it be prevented?

Refeeding syndrome is a potentially fatal but often undiagnosed complication that occurs in severely malnourished patients due to any cause. The aggressive initiation of feeding after prolonged starvation may precipitate numerous metabolic and pathophysiological alterations, leading to severe cardiac, respiratory, hepatic, haematological and neuromuscular complications and even death. (See Chapter 17.)

What are the main complications of parenteral nutrition?

PN should be applied only by experienced medical stuff, as it is associated with several potential risks. First of all, PN is associated with complications related to intravenous access. The establishment and maintenance of PN access may lead to:

- trauma on the central line placement, e.g. carotid puncture or pneumothorax
- thrombophlebitis, especially when PN is provided peripherally
- catheter occlusion and thromboembolism
- air embolism
- infection of sepsis at the catheter site.

These complications can be reduced if the personnel applying the PN are trained and use full aseptic techniques. The possibility of catheter occlusion can be minimised if PN solutions are given from dedicated intravenous catheters and the danger of infection or sepsis can be reduced if changes in catheters and PN bags are performed with strict aseptic techniques.

Apart from the complications associated with intravenous access, PN is associated with metabolic and fluid-related complications. Acute and serious biochemical alterations may be caused by the provision of a large osmolar load to the circulation, resulting in refeeding syndrome. Hyperglycaemia due to diabetes or stress-induced insulin resistance is rather common and should be treated with insulin. PN can also cause fluid imbalances and hepatic disturbances, but the latter are mainly caused by the presence of sepsis or side effects from other drugs rather than by PN itself.

What is hyperalimentation? How can it be prevented?

In the past, in order to reverse catabolism and to maintain the nutritional status of patients, deliberate overfeeding, or hyperalimentation, was initiated. Later research on hyperalimentation, though, came to the conclusion that the provision of PN that exceeds the patient's needs increases the risk of several complications. It can cause uraemia, hyperglycaemia, hyperlipidaemia, fatty liver (hepatic steatosis), hypercapnia (especially with the provision of excessive amounts of carbohydrates) and fluid overload. Overfeeding can be prevented by not exceeding the patients' nutritional needs and by measuring their basal metabolic rate by indirect calorimetry. As it is probable that at least some of the risks of PN are actually related to overfeeding, some organisations now recommend deliberate underfeeding (aiming to meet roughly 85% of a patient's nutritional requirements).

How can hyperglycaemia be prevented? What is the main complication caused by untreated hyperglycaemia in critically ill patients receiving total parenteral nutrition?

Hyperglycaemia is a rather common complication in critically ill patients. It can be caused by hyperalimentation or by insulin resistance to the stress response. A proportion of all hospitalised patients either has diabetes or impaired glucose tolerance (pre-diabetic state). Hyperglycaemia may lead to glycosuria (an excessive excretion of water by the kidney), resulting in hyperosmolar dehydration, which may be fatal for the patient if it remains untreated.

To prevent hyperglycaemia, strict glucose control has been shown to be of great importance, as it has a significant positive impact on mortality in critically ill patients. It has been suggested that the prevention of hyperglycaemia should be the aim of treatment in the first three days of nutritional support (glucose <8.3 mmol/l or 150 mg/dl) and then if the patient is still critically ill to aim for tighter control (4.4–6.1 mmol/l or 80–110 mg/dl).

What additions can be made in parenteral nutrition solutions?

Apart from micronutrient and vitamin additions to the parenteral solutions, some medications can be added. The medications most commonly added to the feed are insulin, in order to avoid hyperglycaemia, and antacids, to avoid gastroduodenal stress ulceration. In order to avoid incompatibilities with the components of the feed, caution must be exercised when adding other medications. More specifically, diuretics, vasopressors, antibiotics and narcotics can be added to the feed, provided that they are compatible with the solution's contents.

What is the role of parenteral nutrition pre- and postoperatively?

Pre-operatively, PN may improve the surgical outcome in several malnourished patients. In well-nourished or moderately malnourished patients, it has not been shown to have beneficial effects, as the risk of complication outweighs any potential benefit.

Postoperatively, PN should be initiated in malnourished patients when enteral nutrition cannot be initiated for a period of 5–7 days. In well-nourished patients, PN should be considered only if the oral or enteral nutrition will not be possible for an extended period.

Is total parenteral nutrition indicated for patients with acute pancreatitis?

Severe acute pancreatitis interferes with nutrient digestion and absorption and is associated with protein catabolism, metabolic instability and increased nutritional requirement. Pancreatitis by itself is not an indication for TPN. A recently published meta-analysis has shown that TPN, as compared with enteral nutrition, significantly increases the risk of infective complications, increases the likelihood of a surgical intervention (to control pancreatic infection) and increases the length of hospital stay.

In patients with mild acute pancreatitis, nutritional support has a minimal benefit as most of them are usually well nourished and can tolerate the necessary period of 5–7 days for pancreatic rest without oral or enteral feeding.

Chapter 18

Moreover, even in severe cases of pancreatitis, enteral feeding through a nasoenteric or jejunal tube has been shown to be effective and safe. PN should be reserved for patients with severe pancreatitis who cannot tolerate enteral nutrition, who have an exacerbation of their disease with enteral feeding and for those about to undergo pancreatic surgery if they have severe signs of malnutrition. Moreover, TPN may be needed in necrotic pancreatitis, pancreatic abscesses and pancreatic pseudocysts.

What are the three-in-one parenteral formulations?

Ready-to-use bags for PN, containing protein, glucose and lipid in a bag with separate sterile champers, which are perforated and mixed before hanging, are called 'three-in-one solutions'. These bags of PN are usually more easy to use for the nursing staff, lower in cost and are preferred to making up individual parenteral solutions. However, these solutions are not flexible and cannot cover the needs of individual patients.

What is transitional nutrition? What is the safest way to pass from parenteral to enteral nutrition?

Transitional nutrition is the moving from one type of feeding to the other, with multiple feeding methods used simultaneously. Transitional nutrition can be from:

- *Parenteral to enteral nutrition*: initially, enteral nutrition should be introduced gradually, at a low rate (30–40 ml/hour) to establish GI tolerance. PN should be decreased, to keep the prescribed nutritional provision. As enteral nutrition will increase gradually, PN will decrease accordingly and can be discontinued when patients achieve 75% of their nutritional needs through enteral nutrition.
- *Parenteral to oral nutrition*: oral intake should be monitored and PN should be discontinued when 75% of the patient's needs are covered by oral intake. The disadvantage of this process is that it is less predictable as it is strongly dependent on the patient's appetite and motivation.

'Transitional nutrition' can also refer to the movement of enteral to oral feeding, for enterally fed patients who are able and have the desire to eat.

What are the indications for home parenteral nutrition? How should it be administered?

Home parenteral nutrition (HPN) is the provision of nutritional support parenterally, usually through a tunnelled catheter, in patients with chronic intestinal failure, where oral or enteral feeding is either ineffective or unsafe. If the intestinal failure is considered irreversible, the feasibility of HPN should be considered. The most common indication of HPN is short bowel syndrome;

Chapter 18

a cyclical provision of the feed (e.g. feed infused overnight) is often advised as it permits patients' mobility through the day and may reduce PN hepatic complications.

Patients receiving HPN should be supported by a coordinated multidisciplinary team, consisting of surgeons, specialist nutrition nurses, dieticians, GPs, pharmacists and district and/or homecare company nurses.

Further reading

American Dietetic Association (2000) *Manual of Clinical Dietetics*, (6th edn). American Dietetic Association, Chicago.

American Society for Parenteral and Enteral Nutrition (ASPEN) Board of Directors and Clinical Guidelines Task Force (2002) Guidelines for the use of parenteral and enteral nutrition in adult and pediatric patients. *Journal of Parenteral and Enteral Nutrition* **26**(suppl.): 1–137SA.

De Beer K, Michael S, Thacker M *et al.* (2008) Diabetic ketoacidosis and hyperglycaemic hyperosmolar syndrome: Clinical guidelines. *Nursing in Critical Care* **13**(1): 5–11.

Gillanders L, Angstmann K, Ball P *et al.* (2008) AuSPEN clinical practice guideline for home parenteral nutrition patients in Australia and New Zealand. *Nutrition* **24**(10): 998–1012.

Ioannidis O, Lavrentieva A, Botsios D (2008) Nutrition support in acute pancreatitis. *Journal of Pancreas* **9**(4): 375–90.

Koretz RL, Lipman TO, Klein S (2001) American Gastrenterological Association technical review on parenteral nutrition. *Gastroenterology* **121**(4): 970–1001.

Mahan KL, Escott-Stump S (1999) *Krause's Food, Nutrition and Diet Therapy*, (10th edn). WB Saunders, Philadelphia.

Marik PE, Zaloga GP (2004) Meta-analysis of parenteral nutrition versus enteral nutrition in patients with acute pancreatitis. *British Medical Journal* **328**(7453): 1407.

Meier R, Beglinger C, Layer P *et al.* (2002) ESPEN Guidelines on Nutrition in acute pancreatitis: European Society of Parenteral and Enteral Nutrition. *Clinical Nutrition* **21**(2): 173–83.

National Institute for Health and Clinical Excellence (2006) *Nutrition support in adults: Oral nutrition support, enteral tube feeding and parenteral nutrition* (Clinical Guideline 32). NICE, London, http://www.nice.org.uk/nicemedia/pdf/cg032fullguideline.pdf.

Veterans Affairs Total Parenteral Nutrition Cooperative Study Group (1991) Perioperative total parenteral nutrition in surgical patients. *New England Journal of Medicine* **325**(8): 525–32.

Chapter 19

Food Allergy

Meropi Kontogianni

What are the main differences between food allergy and non-allergic food intolerance?

'Food allergy' refers to specific reactions that result from an abnormal immunological response to a food and which can be severe and life-threatening and triggered by minute amounts of the allergen. Conversely, 'non-allergic food intolerance' refers to reactions to food that can result from a number of causes, none of which is mediated by the immune system (e.g. pharmacological effects, enzyme deficiencies, irritant and toxic effects). Owing to their variable aetiology, their effects can be acute and severe, although rarely life-threatening, but they are usually chronic and diffuse. Unlike food allergy, relatively large amounts of a food are usually necessary for adverse effects to occur.

What are the main types of food allergy and how are they clinically presented?

There are two major classes of food allergic reactions: immunoglobulin E (IgE) mediated and non-IgE mediated. The former are generally present soon after ingestion and thus easy to investigate and diagnose. They can be more violent than non-IgE mediated reactions and can even lead to death through anaphylaxis in severe cases. Non-IgE mediated reactions are often presented later and can be more subtle and often an important cause of ill health. Food-allergic reactions are generally divided into those of early onset (within minutes to an hour after food ingestion), which also tend to be IgE mediated, and those of late onset (taking hours or days), which are in general non-IgE mediated. Early-onset manifestations often include wheezing, urticaria, angioedema, rashes, vomiting and anaphylaxis, whereas late-onset symptoms include diarrhoea, abdominal pain, allergic rhinitis, atopic eczema, food-sensitive enteropathy or food-sensitive colitis, protein-losing enteropathy and constipation.

What foods are known to cause immunologically mediated reactions?

Common foods that can cause an allergic reaction include:

- peanuts and tree nuts (e.g. hazelnut, Brazil nut, walnut)
- milk (cow's, goat's, sheep's)
- soya
- fish
- shellfish
- eggs
- seeds (especially sesame and caraway)
- fruits (especially apples, peaches, plums, cherries, bananas, citrus fruits)
- herbs and spices (especially mustard, paprika and coriander).

However, the most common allergies, according to the frequency they occur, are:

- *in children:* cow's milk, egg, soya, peanut, tree nuts, fish and crustaceans
- *in adults:* peanut, tree nuts, crustaceans, fish and egg.

The processing of food may also affect its allergenicity. For example, the allergenicity of many fruits may be greatly reduced by cooking, and that of eggs, milk and some fish may be attenuated. It is also possible that the boiling, but not the roasting, of peanuts may lessen their allergenicity. On the other hand, the thermal processing of food may lead to the formation of allergens that are not present in raw foods. This may be attributed to changes in the shape of protein molecules and the revealing of previously hidden epitopes.

Moreover, allergies to 'new' foods commonly emerge as these foods are introduced to a new population. Thus, kiwi fruit allergy has become a significant problem in the UK in recent years. In addition, novel food proteins from genetically modified organisms or from new manufacturing processes applied to existing foods could carry a risk of food allergy.

How can food allergy be diagnosed?

The diagnosis of IgE mediated food allergy is usually based on a patient's medical history and confirmed by the results of one or more specific investigations, including skin tests, blood tests [radioallergosorbent (RAST) tests, enzyme-linked immunosorbent assay (ELISA)], response to dietary restriction (single exclusion diet, multiple-food exclusion diet, elemental and protein hydrolysate formula diet) and sometimes by oral challenge tests. The confirmation of non-IgE mediated (delayed) food allergy is more difficult to achieve and is largely based on dietary restriction and oral challenge tests.

How can a dietitian contribute to the management of food allergies?

The management of allergic diseases is recognised as an area of specialisation and should ideally be carried out by a clinical immunology and allergy team, which would include medical expertise from the fields of respiratory diseases, dermatology, gastroenterology and immunology and the specialist skills of dietitians and nurses. This team should identify and completely avoid the offending allergen or allergens. Specialist dietetic guidance is essential to ensure that

- all potential sources of the allergen are avoided
- the effects of the exclusion diet on the intake of other nutrients and overall dietary balance are minimised.

This is especially important for infants and children, and in the event that the excluded food is a major nutritional contributor (e.g. milk), because alternative sources of nutrients should be provided. Dietitians should also provide written guidance on the foods or types of foods that must be avoided, foods or types of foods that may need to be avoided, which is determined from ingredients lists of manufactured foods, and foods or types of foods that can be safely eaten. Dietary advice in order to prevent potential nutritional inadequacies is also crucial. Moreover, dietitians should teach their patients to:

- carefully check all ingredient labels
- learn other names of the food responsible for the allergy
- exercise caution when eating out since restaurant staff are not always aware of specific menu ingredients or how food is prepared
- be careful when eating food that is packaged in multi-packs with other foods: while one product may be considered safe, there is a risk of cross-contamination because products may leak or become unwrapped.

Further reading

Barth B, Furuta GT (2004) These FADs are here to stay: Clinicopathological patterns of food allergic diseases. *Gastroenterology* **126**(5): 1481–2.

Committee on Toxicity of Chemicals in Food, Consumer Products and the Environment (2000) *Adverse Reactions to Food and Food Ingredients: Report of a working group on food intolerance.* Food Standards Agency, London, http://cot.food.gov.uk/pdfs/adversereactionstofood.pdf.

European Society for Paediatric Gastroenterology and Nutrition Working Group for the Diagnostic Criteria for Food Allergy (1992) Diagnostic criteria for food allergy with predominantly intestinal symptoms. *Journal of Pediatric Gastroenterology Nutrition* **14**(1): 108–12.

Johansson SG, Bieber T, Dahl R *et al.* (2004) Revised nomenclature for allergy for global use: Report of the Nomenclature Review Committee of the World Allergy

Chapter 19

Organization, October 2003. *Journal of Allergy and Clinical Immunology* **113**(5): 832–6.

Lack G (2008) Clinical practice: Food allergy. *New England Journal of Medicine* **359**(12): 1252–60.

Ministry of Agricultural, Fisheries & Food (1997) *Food Allergy and Other Unpleasant Reactions to Food.* MAFF, London.

Index

Keep up with critical fields

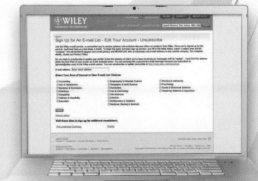
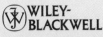